GRASSLAND BEEF PRODUCTION

CURRENT TOPICS IN VETERINARY MEDICINE AND ANIMAL SCIENCE

GRASSLAND BEEF PRODUCTION

A Seminar in the CEC Programme of Coordination of Research on Beef Production, held at the Centre for European Agricultural Studies, Wye College (University of London), Ashford, Kent, UK, July 25–27, 1983

Sponsored by the Commission of the European Communities, Directorate-General for Agriculture, Coordination of Agricultural Research

Edited by

W. Holmes
Wye College, Ashford, Kent, UK

1984 **MARTINUS NIJHOFF PUBLISHERS**
a member of the KLUWER ACADEMIC PUBLISHERS GROUP
BOSTON / THE HAGUE / DORDRECHT / LANCASTER
for
THE COMMISSION OF THE EUROPEAN COMMUNITIES

Distributors

for the United States and Canada: Kluwer Boston, Inc., 190 Old Derby Street, Hingham, MA 02043, USA
for all other countries: Kluwer Academic Publishers Group, Distribution Center, P.O.Box 322, 3300 AH Dordrecht, The Netherlands

Library of Congress Cataloging in Publication Data

ISBN-13: 978-94-009-6026-8   e-ISBN-13: 978-94-009-6024-4
DOI: 10.1007/978-94-009-6024-4

Book information

Publication arranged by: Commission of the European Communities, Directorate-General Information Market and Innovation, Luxembourg
Typed and prepared for reproduction by: Joy E. Rees and Hilary C. Marsh, Wye College, Ashford, Kent, UK

Copyright/legal notice

P R E F A C E

In the agriculture of the western areas of the European Community grassland is often the most appropriate crop and when milk production is adequate this grassland should be converted into beef or sheep products.

Accordingly the Commission of the European Communities encouraged the organisation of a seminar on beef production from grassland which was held at Wye College (University of London), Ashford, Kent, UK in July, 1983.

This book contains the text of 22 papers and posters presented at the seminar together with a summary of the final discussion.

The papers described the background to beef production in several European countries and outlined methods of production for beef animals fed mainly on grass both for cattle derived from dairy herds and from single suckler herds. Particular attention was paid to the additional contribution possible from bull beef production and to methods of relating animal production to predicted herbage production. The objectives in breeding for beef production were considered and it was concluded that performance tests on beef bulls should be designed so that they corresponded closely with the conditions under which commercial beef cattle would be produced. Experimental methods applicable to the conduct of beef experiments on grassland were also considered.

The summary includes suggestions for further investigational or development work.

CONTENTS

AGRICULTURAL RESEARCH CO-ORDINATION IN THE EUROPEAN COMMUNITY

W.F. Raymond

Visiting Professor, Wye College, University of London, formerly Chief Scientist (Agriculture), Ministry of Agriculture, Fisheries and Food, UK

The 1957 Treaty of Rome recognised that, for the European Communities to develop their full potential in science and technology, close collaboration would be needed between the research services of the individual member states. To that end the Directorate General for Science Research and Development, DG XII,was set up to co-ordinate the national research programmes in a number of key subjects such as energy,raw materials, environment and information science. Exceptionally however the co-ordination of research in agriculture was made the responsibility of the Directorate General for Agriculture, DG VI.

Apart from some collaboration in veterinary subjects there had been in fact little activity in agricultural research until 1972. In that year the Commission set up the Standing Committee for Agricultural Research (SCAR). This is composed of senior research directors and administrators from the member states, and meets regularly to consult with the Commission on priority subjects for research co-ordination and to advise the Commission in the management of agreed programmes. To date there have been two such programmes, in 1974-78 and 1979-83 and proposals for the third programme, 1984-88, have recently been submitted to the Council of Ministers and to the European Parliament.

The first programme included six subjects, of which two aimed specifically to increase Community production of two commodities, plant proteins and beef, which seemed likely to be in continuing deficit. The Commission thus set up sub-committees (Programme Committees) to advise it and the SCAR on opportunities for improved research collaboration in these subjects. The Beef Programme Committee included experts in different aspects of beef production from each of the member states; I have been fortunate to be the Chairman of this Committee since 1978, when I took over from R.Février of France,who had by then laid excellent guidelines for the programme.

The Committee rapidly identified several subjects which it considered needed more work including the genetics of beef animals; disease, in particular neo-natal disease; nutrition and management of beef cattle, and carcass and meat quality. An Expert Working Group was then set up to give detailed advice on research priorities within each of these subjects. This advice, together with similar advice from Committees dealing with plant proteins, animal effluents, land use etc., then formed the basis of the research programmes undertaken by DG VI.

These programmes have included two main types of activity:

Common action - proposals for research directly related to the objectives of the programme at the request of the Commission are put forward by leading research centres in the member states; approved projects are then jointly funded with the Commission contributing up to 50% of the cost of the research.

Co-ordination activity - the Commission, advised by the Programme Committees and Expert Groups, has organised many seminars and workshops on priority subjects. Some of these have been held in Brussels, but many have been held at important research centres in the member states, with the detailed arrangements being made by scientists at the centres. Visits by Community scientists to other laboratories, for periods ranging from a few days to several weeks, have also been funded by the Commission.

These seminars and workshops have proved of considerable value; the number of participants has generally been restricted to about 30 which has allowed a more informal and detailed discussion than is often possible in larger international meetings, as well as the practical demonstration of new techniques and equipment in laboratories and animal houses.

This present seminar is one of about 100 similar meetings which are being sponsored by the Commission during 1983, within the overall activity of agricultural research co-ordination. Its particular importance is that it links together the themes of two programmes, by examining ways of improving the efficiency and reducing the costs of beef production and at the same time reducing the need for feeding supplementary plant proteins, by making better use of grazed and conserved grass. As with many earlier seminars, the aim is for the papers and the main conclusions of the meeting to be published as a book by the Commission.

This is in fact one of the last seminars that will be held specifically on beef production, for beef is not one of the priority subjects in the new programme that the Commission is due to start in 1984, though aspects closely related to beef production will be included in the proposed programmes on animal pathology, animal reproduction, animal welfare and food quality. However as a result of the many meetings that have been held during the last ten years, Community research workers dealing with beef production now know of the work of their colleagues in the other member states on a much more detailed and personal basis than has ever before been possible; our aim now must be to continue and further strengthen this most valuable collaboration.

TECHNICAL AND ECONOMIC BACKGROUND TO BEEF PRODUCTION IN BRITAIN

W. Holmes

Wye College, University of London

Beef production is an important sector of British agriculture. In financial terms it accounts for 17% of total agricultural output and is exceeded only by arable products (24%) and milk (22%). Sheep, the other grazing livestock, account for just over 4%. In the EEC of 9 the corresponding figures are 15% for beef and 19% for milk while sheep production is of only minor importance.

Geographical and economic factors influence the choice of agricultural enterprises. Climate and topography favour arable production only in the East of Britain and much of the country is suited only to grass production. Dairy farming occurs in the more favoured grassland areas and beef production is found in the less favoured grass areas and is also integrated, in some regions, with arable farming.

Some comparative data on cattle and beef cattle populations and production in the EEC are in Table 1. Only France, UK, Ireland and Greece

TABLE 1   Data on EEC cattle, 1981

Country	Total cattle M	Total cows M	Dairy cows % of total cows	Average beef carcase weights kg	Average herd sizes	
					all cattle	dairy cows
Germany	14.9	5.6	97	296	29	13
France	22.8	9.7	71	323	35	15
Italy	8.9	3.8	80	263	13	6
Netherlands	5.0	2.4	100	285	62	36
Belgium	2.8	1.1	88	341	39	18
Luxembourg	0.2	0.08	85	286	62	24
UK	13.0	4.7	70	265	77	56
Ireland	5.8	1.9	78	269	33	15
Denmark	2.9	1.1	93	230	50	26
Greece	0.8	0.36	64	216	6	3

From:
MMB, 1982 Facts and Figures;   EEC 1982

have large proportions of beef breeding cattle. Otherwise beef is derived primarily from the dairy herd. In Britain the number of beef cows rose rapidly after 1946 to peak at 1.9M in 1975 but has since declined to 1.4M. Home production of beef increased from 0.55Mt in 1946 to 1.2Mt in 1975. It is now just over 1Mt and provides over 90% of total consumption.

The level of protein supplies for the human population and changes in consumption of meats and cheese in Britain are shown in Table 2. Beef consumption is stable or declining slightly, sheep meat has fallen while pork and poultry meat consumption have increased considerably.

Beef production is seldom the major enterprise on British farms. It is commonly combined with sheep farming on grassland or on grassland/arable farms and sometimes occurs jointly with dairy farming. Only 7000 herds exceed 50 breeding cows. As in much of Europe therefore British beef is mainly derived from dairy cows. The Meat and Livestock Commission(1983)

TABLE 2   Changes in the average British diet

	1960	1979
Protein g/d	84.5	83.4
Animal protein g/d	49.7	51.5
Meat kg/an	56.2	58.5
Beef	21.3	22.0
Sheep	11.4	7.1
Pork	8.6	12.3
Bacon	11.3	10.7
Poultry	5.6	13.2
Cheese	4.4	5.9

Ashby, A.W. (1982).

estimates that 43% of British beef production is from steers and heifers bred in the dairy herd, 19% from culled dairy cows, 34% from beef breeds and the remaining 4% from cattle of beef type imported from Ireland.Because of prejudice by butchers, farmers and consumers entire bulls are seldom retained for beef production in Britain.

There have been important changes in breed preference which are illustrated in Table 3. Before 1940 the cattle population was dominated by the Dairy Shorthorn, a dual purpose breed. It has now virtually disappeared and over 80% of our 3.2M dairy cows are of the Friesian breed.

The Friesian therefore makes a large contribution to British beef production. Most of the pure beef herds are bred naturally so that Table 3 based on artificial insemination data gives only a partial guide although bull licensing figures were in agreement. The table illustrates the increasing popularity of the Charolais, introduced to UK about 1960 and the Limousin, introduced in 1970. Use of these breeds has increased at the expense of Hereford and Angus and the local beef breeds of which the Sussex is an example, and which include Devon, Galloway and Welsh Black. Colour marking particularly shown by Hereford and Charolais has economic importance. Much comparative information has been assembled in Britain on

TABLE 3   Changes in breed preferences in England and Wales

	Matings in the dairy herd		
	1976-77	%	1981-82
Aberdeen Angus	4.0		3.1
Charolais	4.9		6.8
Hereford	20.5		17.7
Limousin	0.5		4.1
Simmental	1.2		1.0
Sussex	0.3		0.1
Other beef breeds	1.8		1.2
Total beef	33.2		34.0
Friesian/Holstein	61.4		62.0
Other dairy breeds	4.8		3.6

the relative merits of beef breeds (e.g. Limousin and Simmental Tests Steering Committee, 1977, Southgate 1982) and this information is now available in Allen and Kilkenny (1980) and in advisory literature. About 62% of all artificial inseminations are with Friesian/Holstein bulls. Canadian Holsteins which are increasingly used in Friesian herds will probably have adverse effects on beef production (More O'Ferrall,1982)

Systems of British beef production

British beef production methods include suckler (cow-calf) systems and dairy bred systems. The major systems and their dependence on concentrate feeding are listed in Table 4. Increased concentrate feeding is associated with reduced carcase weight. Similar figures are given by Kilkenny and Dench (1981) who also point out the large proportion of the costs of production (35 to 60%) attributable to concentrates in British beef production. Green and Baker (1981) estimated that concentrates provided 21% of all ME required for British beef production in 1976. Comparable figures for the dairy herd were 40% and for sheep and horses 3%. The wide difference in feed costs between concentrates (1.0 - 1.5p/MJ,ME), conserved forage (c.0.6p/MJ) and grazed grass (c.0.3p/MJ) explains the continuing interest in the potential contribution of grass to beef production.

TABLE 4   Typical concentrate allocation per head and proportion of
metabolizable energy from concentrates for British
beef systems

	Concentrates kg/head	Proportion of ME %
Suckler systems		
Suckler cow (per year)	250	10
15 month autumn calves	900	10
24 month spring calves	700	20
Dairy beef systems		
Cereal beef	1800	95
15 month grass cereal beef	1200	50
18 month grass cereal beef	1100	40
24 month grass beef	1000	25
36 month grass beef	600	10

The figures for gross margin (financial output less variable costs) in Table 5 illustrate the differences between systems of production although differences in common costs are also important.

Better use of grassland may result from the development and application of targets for appropriate stocking rates (e.g. Holmes, 1968; 1982; Allen & Kilkenny, 1980),the rational use of nitrogenous fertilizers which can yield 1 kg liveweight gain per kg nitrogen applied and from the skilled utilization of supplementary feeds as green forages, stored forages or concentrates.

TABLE 5   Five year average gross margins in beef production,MLC 1983

	Average gross margins	
	£ per head	£ per ha
Cereal beef	51	−
Maize silage beef	160	1052
Grass silage beef	154	1141
18 month beef	196	613
20-24 month beef	210	443
Lowland suckler herds	149	283
Upland suckler herds	186	223
Grass finishing of store cattle	59	330

Biological efficiency

All forms of beef production are relatively costly because of their low biological efficiency. Some values are given in Table 6 and other data may be seen in Holmes, 1977 and Spedding, Walsingham and Hoxey, 1981. The contrast with the milking cow is striking. Pigs and poultry are also more efficient than beef animals but are dependent on high quality feeds while sheep are of a comparable order of efficiency to beef cattle. Beef and sheep can of course utilise land of low agricultural potential.

TABLE 6   Calculated efficiencies of feed conversion %*

	ME	GE	CP
Suckler systems			
Rear beef heifers to 2 years,slaughter	8.0	4.4	10.3
Rear heifer, calve at 2 years, slaughter cow at 3 years and calf at 15 months	6.0	3.3	7.4
Rear beef cow, rear 8 calves in 9 years to 15 months, slaughter cow	3.7	2.0	4.6
Dairy beef systems			
12 month cereal	10.0	7.0	13.0
15 month grass cereal	9.2	5.6	11.7
18 month grass cereal	8.5	5.0	10.6
24 month grass	7.1	4.1	8.3
Dairy systems			
Milk cow, 4 lactations of 5000 kg milk	22.0	13.2	27.0

* Edible energy as a percentage of metabolizable energy (ME) or gross energy (GE) edible protein as a percentage of crude protein, in feed

With both sheep and cattle the high maintenance cost of a dam of low prolificacy is a major limitation to efficiency of production. As Fig. 1 shows, doubling the number of young reared would raise productivity (and efficiency) by approximately 50%. The high annual feed requirement also suggests that longevity is not very important in a beef herd and indeed Table 6 indicates that once bred heifers are more efficient than cows producing a succession of calves.

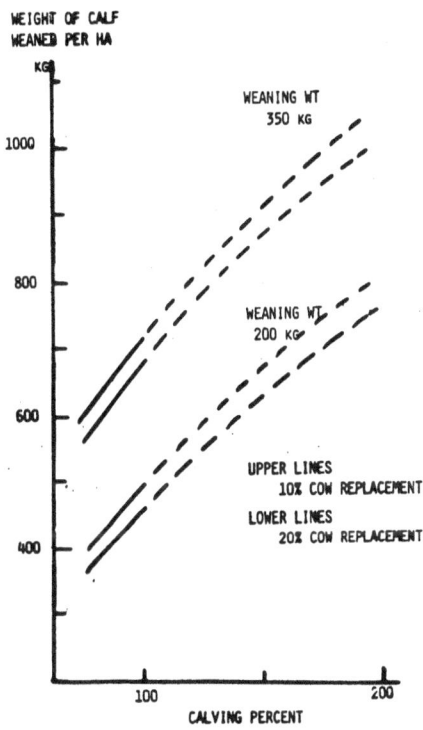

Fig. 1 The influence of calving percentage, weaning weight and cow replacement rate on potential weight of calf weaned per ha

The future

The value of animal enterprises to the farmer depends both on their biological efficiency and on the level of prices, and high prices for beef relative to other meats and to feed costs can justify beef production.

The demand for beef will probably remain high since it is the preferred meat for many consumers, but both high price and high fat content in the meat could reduce demand. Measures to cheapen production and to reduce fat content are therefore required.

These measures will include:

a) improvements in prolificacy, resulting from good husbandry, genetic selection and possibly from physiological manipulation

b) enhanced growth, a result of genetic selection, appropriate choice of breed, the appropriate use of growth promoting substances and better feeding

c) cheapness of production by more rapid finishing and by the greater use of cheaper but high quality forage based diets

d) reduction of fat content of carcasses by the use of bulls, a reduction in the use of cereal concentrates and slaughtering at an earlier stage of development.

It is the purpose of this seminar to explore some of these possibilities.

REFERENCES

Allen, D.M. and Kilkenny, J.B. 1980. Planned beef production.   Granada: London.

Ashby, A.W. 1982. Our changing diet, lessons for farmers. Agricultural Progress **57** 3-12.

EEC 1982. The agricultural situation in the Community. CEC, Brussels

Green,J.O. and Baker, R.D. 1981. Classification, distribution and productivity of UK grasslands. In: Grassland in the British Economy. Ed. J.L. Jollans, CAS Paper No.10, Centre for Agricultural Strategy, Reading

Holmes, W. 1968. The use of nitrogen in the management of pasture for cattle. Herb. Abstr. **38** 265-277

Holmes, W. 1977. Choosing between animals. Phil. Trans R.Soc. Lond.B. **281** 121-137

Holmes, W. 1982. Grass, its production and utilisation. Ed.W. Holmes. Blackwells: Oxford

Kilkenny, J.B. and Dench, J.A.L. 1981. The role of grassland in beef production. In: Grassland in the British Economy. Ed. J.L. Jollans. CAS Paper No.10, Centre for Agricultural Strategy, Reading

Limousin Simmental Tests Steering Committee, 1977. An evaluation of Limousin and Simmental Bulls in Britain. HMSO: London

MLC, 1983. Beef Yearbook. Meat and Livestock Commission, Milton Keynes, UK

MMB 1982. EEC Dairy Facts and Figures, Milk Marketing Board, Thames Ditton

More O'Ferrall, G.J. (Ed) 1982. Beef production from different dairy breeds and dairy breed crosses. Martinus Nijhoff:The Hague,Netherlands

Southgate, J.R. 1982. The current practice of commercial cross breeding in the UK with particular reference to the effects of breed choice. In: Beef production from different dairy breeds and dairy breed crosses. (Ed. G.J. More O'Ferrall) Martinus Nijhoff: The Hague,Netherlands

Spedding, C.R.W., Walsingham,J.M. and Hoxey, A.M. 1981. Biological efficiency in agriculture. Academic Press:London

FRENCH BEEF PRODUCTION SYSTEMS FROM GRASSLAND

by D. Micol and C. Béranger

Institut National de la Recherche Agronomique, Centre de Recherches
Zootechniques et Vétérinaires, Theix, 63122 Ceyrat, France

Beef production in France originates from different types of animals produced more or less intensively. Approximately two thirds of the beef produced comes from the dairy herd and one third from the beef cow herd. Most of the steers and heifers, and recently a small proportion of the young bulls are reared principally on grass. Intensively reared young bulls contribute only about 14% of beef produced (Table 1) and one quarter of these are from the beef herd, and use grass during the suckling period. Dry culled cows are also often finished on pasture.

TABLE 1   Distribution pattern of beef slaughtered in France during 1980 (estimation according to the types of animal from dairy or beef herd)

	Dairy breed				Beef breed				Total
	Number ('000)	p 100	Carcass weight (kg)	Total weight ('000 t)	Number ('000)	p 100	Carcass weight (kg)	Total weight ('000 t)	Weight ('000 t)
Young bulls	440	14	330	145	144	11	380	58	203
Steers	690	21	345	238	220	18	415	91	329
Heifers	420	13	275	116	360	28	310	112	227
Cows	1655	52	280	463	538	43	310	167	630
Total	3205	100	300	962	1262	100	338	428	1389

A Faucon d'après SCEES et GEB, 1981

Beef production from steers and heifers is developed principally in the pasture areas of the North-West, North-East and Middle East of France, and some fattening cattle remaining on the arable plains to the North of Paris. (Fig. 1). Beef cow herds are mainly located on grassland areas in the South Loire Valley and in the West Rhone Valley and particularly in the centre of France. (Fig. 2)

Various types of animals are produced from both beef and dairy breeds according to age, weight at slaughter and shape of growth curve. In traditional systems the growth of steers and heifers is essentially

12

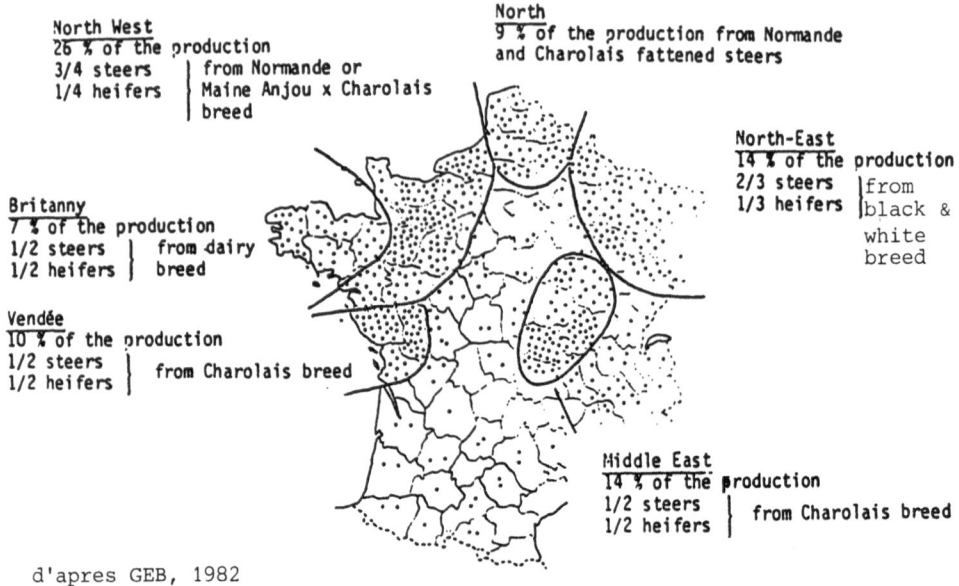

North West
26 % of the production
3/4 steers | from Normande or
1/4 heifers | Maine Anjou x Charolais
            | breed

North
9 % of the production from Normande
and Charolais fattened steers

Britanny
7 % of the production
1/2 steers | from dairy
1/2 heifers | breed

North-East
14 % of the production
2/3 steers | from
1/3 heifers | black &
             white
             breed

Vendée
10 % of the production
1/2 steers | from Charolais breed
1/2 heifers |

Middle East
14 % of the production
1/2 steers | from Charolais breed
1/2 heifers |

d'apres GEB, 1982

Fig. 1 Areas of beef production from steers and heifers in France

achieved on grass after low winter gains. Semi-intensive systems are also
mainly based on the utilisation of grazed and conserved grass (Fig. 3).

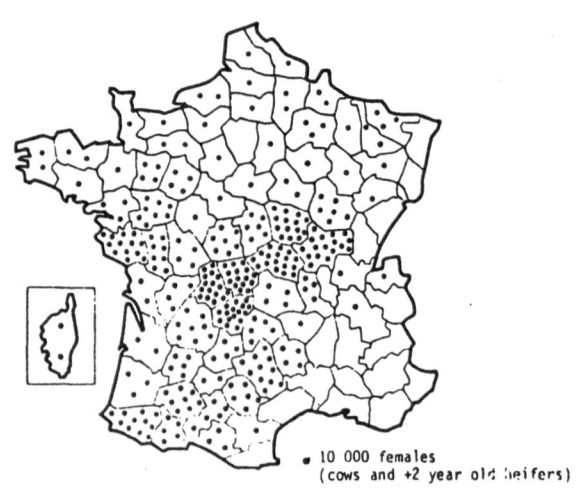

● 10 000 females
(cows and +2 year old heifers)

Fig. 2 Distribution of beef cow herds in France (1977)

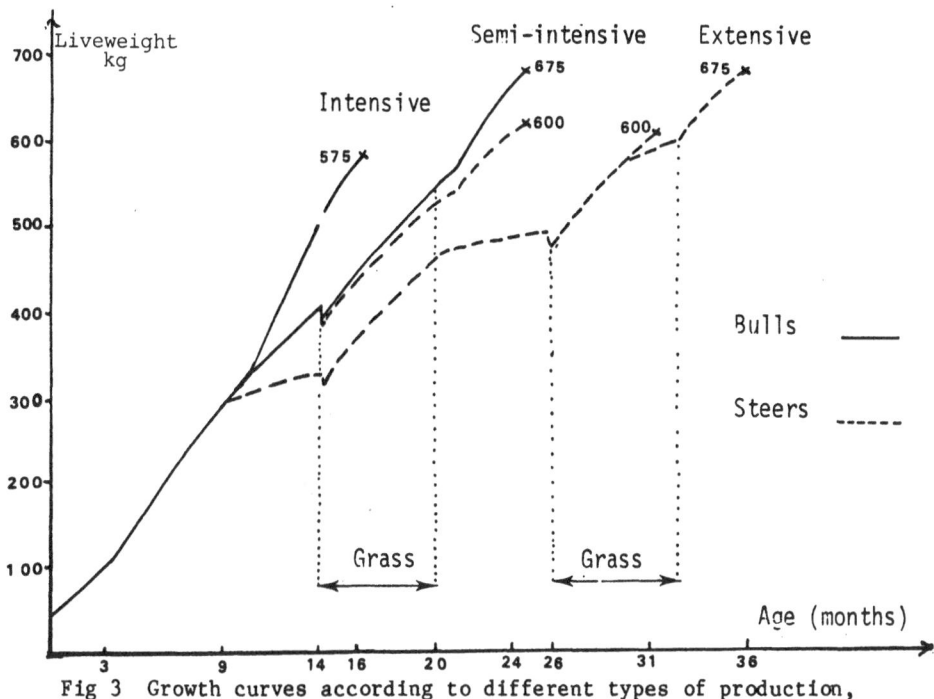

Fig 3   Growth curves according to different types of production, example taken from Charolais crossbred animals

The average stocking rate is rather low per ha of forage (grassland + forage crop) in areas where steers or heifers are produced, (except on certain western areas) as well as in the beef cow areas (Fig. 4).   Given that the average value for the country is around 1.12 U.G.B./ha S.F.P. (*) the higher stocking rates are found in areas of dairy production.   In beef producing areas the higher stocking rates are often on farms growing forage maize and stocking rates on pasture are therefore often very low. Improvements in grassland utilisation as well in animal performance are possible in many situations.

* U.G.B.: Cattle unit corresponding to 3,000 feed units/year, i.e. a dairy cow of 550 kg LW producing 3,000 kg of milk.
  S.F.P.: Total area of grassland and forage crops (feed from other crops excluded).

IMPROVEMENT OF GRASSLAND UTILISATION IN BEEF PRODUCTION

Under traditional production systems most steers and heifers are finished on grass, especially by grazing permanent pasture.   As it is necessary to reach a certain level of gain to obtain sufficient fattening from grass only, some consider that it is not possible to increase the stocking rate on pasture for finishing steers or heifers.   During the growing period, steers and heifers often graze the poorest pastures or more

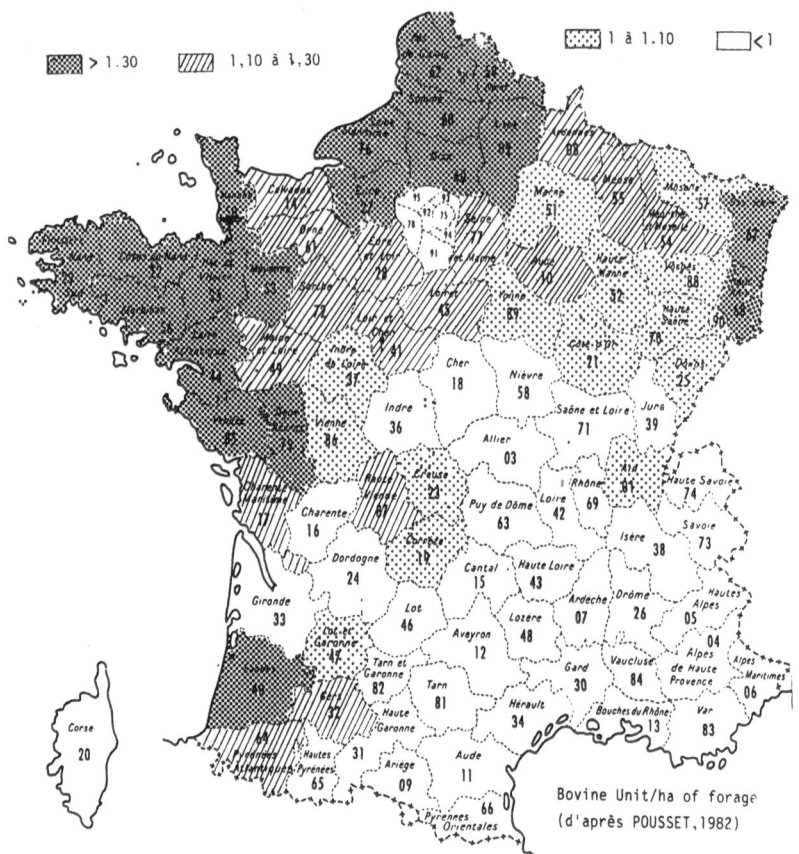

Fig.4 Distribution of stocking rate in France (bovine unit/ha forage)

distant paddocks and their intensification is consequently of low priority. Most conserved grass is cut as hay, giving too late a regrowth for optimal adjustment of stocking rate between the spring and summer period. These factors together with the low levels of nitrogen fertilisation which are common on pastures for beef production explain the low stocking rate.

Many experiments carried out at the INRA farm at Le Pin-au-Haras, Normandy, from 1960 to 1975, have shown that 2 to 3 year old steers can be finished on sown or permanent pastures with a high stocking rate and a high level of beef production per hectare. In oceanic climatic conditions on clay soils,rye grass pastures receiving 150-200 kg Nitrogen/ha,yielded 10 t DM/ha of available grass to grazing steers during 170-180 days. With a "put and take system" the optimum stocking rate was 4.9 steers/ha (2,600 kg liveweight/ha) which produced 820 kg of live weight gain/ha and allowed 84% of the steers to be finished on pasture (Fig. 5).

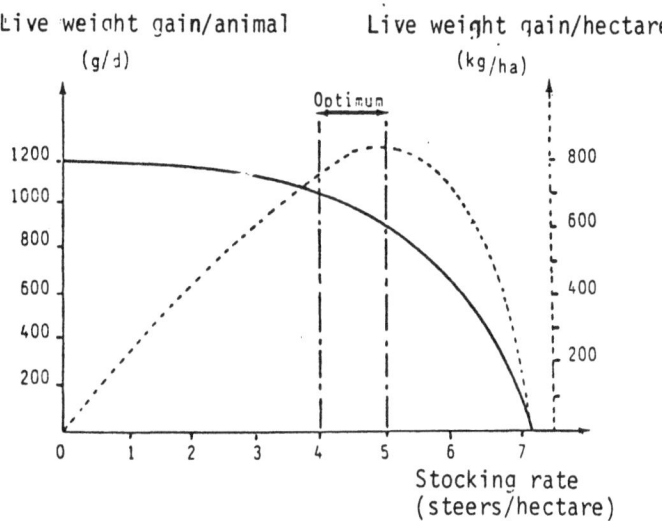

Fig. 5   Effect of stocking rate on beef production from steers
          fattened on grass (INRA - le Pin au Haras)

Under such conditions a stocking rate of 4.5 steers/ha (6 steers/ha in
spring and 3 during summer) can be recommended with the probability of
finishing without concentrate. A good grazing management system is needed
and rotational grazing on 10-12 paddocks, staying 4-5 days in each paddock,
is recommended to attain from 60 to 80% efficiency of grazing.

Similar results may be obtained with younger growing cattle, under
similar grazing conditons. Young animals do not however eat sufficient
grass to attain the same growth rate as 2 year old steers. If the same
stocking rate (in liveweight/ha) is imposed, the greater number of cattle
compensates for the lower rate of gain per animal so that the live weight
gain per hectare is similar for the two types of animals (Béranger, 1977).

Using similar grazing management and lower nitrogen fertilisation
(80-100 kg N/ha) on hill pasture, producing around 5 t DM/ha of available
grass, it is possible to produce 300-350 kg of liveweight gain/ha in
140-150 days with growing heifers, without any conservation (Table 2).
Average gain was 700-900 g/day which is rather good with this type of
animal.

By increasing stocking rate during the early season by cutting
approximately half of the area, it is possible to produce similar live
weight gains/ha, plus 1.5 t of hay, without decreasing significantly
individual liveweight gain (Table 2). At the Le Pin-au-Haras farm, when

TABLE 2   Production of hill pastures grazed by heifers
with or without cutting

	Marcenat 15-1100 m	Laqueuille 63-1200 m	Laqueuille 63-1200 m	Laqueuille 63-1200 m
No years	5	4	3	3
Area (ha)	72	16	8	8
Grazing method	6 paddocks	4 paddocks	4+2 paddocks	continuous grazing
Cutting	None	None	Hay	Hay
Nitrogen fertilization (kg N/ha)	100	80	120	120
Age of heifers (y)	1 and 2	1	1	1
Length of grazing period (d)	150	138	150	150
Stocking rate (kg LW/ha)	1229	1204	1262	1284
Average daily gain (g/d)				
1 year old heifers	826	789	657	662
2 year old heifers	930	-	-	-
Liveweight gain/ha (kg/ha)	357	323	306	309
DM cut for hay (t/ha)	-	-	1.50	1.50

(D. Micol, unpublished data)

the surplus grass was cut during spring for silage, recorded data from 54
experimental grazing groups of young bulls and steers showed a production
per hectare of 560 kg of liveweight gain, plus 1.1 t DM of conserved grass
in 180 days.   A stocking rate of 4.5 animals/ha (i.e. 2,150 kg of
liveweight/ha) with an average daily gain of 700 g was attained for the
total area.

If a slight decline in growth rate is accepted for these animals, a
higher level of intensification may be obtained with this type of system
including early harvesting of excess grass for silage, with higher
fertilisation, stocking rate and speed of rotation. This system is however
complicated and expensive, especially for growing stock.

Intensive continuous grazing, developed in Great Britain in the last
10 years, may simplify grazing management. With high nitrogen supply (300
kg/ha) most of the results obtained in Western Europe showed only a small
decline (-5 -10%) in production of liveweight gain on continuous grazing
versus rotational grazing (Le Du, 1980). At the Le Pin-au-Haras farm, a
comparison over three years led to the same conclusion. It also seems
possible to adopt the continuous grazing method under less intensive
conditions. Three years of experiments in hill pastures in the Auvergne
(Laqueuille 1,200 m altitude) indicated similar production for continuous
versus rotational grazing, with 120 kg nitrogen/ha and 50% of the area cut

once for hay (Table 2). This indicates that simplified grazing methods, based on continuous grazing,using moderate or even low levels of nitrogen fertilisation, could be developed in the future, for the progressive and economic intensification of production from grassland.

IMPROVEMENT OF GRAZING ANIMALS

Beef production from young steers, as in British 18 month grass cereal beef is not possible in France because of the different market requirements for carcass weight and degree of fatness. Intensive production systems therefore depend on the production of young bulls fed indoors after weaning from the suckling herd or after a period of rearing on dairy farms (Fig. 3). In some French trials, young dairy bulls fed intensively were turned out to pasture between 5-8 months and 10-12 months of age for a few months. Compared with bulls fed on maize silage permanently indoors the former needed a longer time to reach the same carcass weight and degree of fatness, without any significant decrease in the cost of feeding. Such a system is rarely used.

The most intensive grassland system which has been studied in France is with steers fattened on grass from 12-14 months to 18-20 months of age (Béranger and Petit, 1971; Béranger, 1977). With the breeds used in France, it is necessary to supplement these animals with at least, 3 kg of grain per day from mid July to slaughter (250-350 kg of grain/animal).

Thus it is possible to produce carcasses weighing 300 kg with a satisfactory fat level (12-14% of separable fat). But this type of production has not developed in France because the carcass weights are low compared with older and heavier steers appearing on the same markets at the same time.

Young bulls produced under the same conditions never fattened on pasture, even with high grain supplementation (500 kg per animal), but always grew faster than similar steers.

To obtain heavy carcasses with sufficient fat, the production of 2 year old bulls, steers or heifers in semi-intensive systems appears to be suitable for efficient grassland utilisation. Under this system animals do not reach their maximum growth potential except during the final 3-5 months finishing period indoors before slaughter. Growth rates must however remain at an adequate level, reaching 500 kg of liveweight for steers and 550 kg for bulls at the beginning of the fattening period in autumn (Fig. 3). This target can be otained with a forage diet during the first winter period which may lead to daily gains of 600 to 1,000 g. On pasture, it is necessary to maintain average gains during the grazing season at a level of 700-900 g/day, which needs good grazing management. A system which integrates grazing with conservation of early cut grass is the most suitable to obtain good animal performance both in summer on pasture and in winter with grass silage.

Such a discontinuous growth curve allows compensatory growth between summer and winter periods especially according to variation of grass silage quality and of grass supply. The experiment reported in Table 3 shows the possibilities of adaptation to variations in feeding without modification of final carcass weight and composition.

Animal performance depends however on sex and breed. Bulls always tend to grow faster than steers (+ 100 to 150 g/day) even under grazing conditions. They produce carcasses weighing 10% more than those of steers and contain 20% more lean (Table 4). It is possible to extend their fattening period and increase the carcass weight without excess of fat deposition, because of their late maturity. The quality of the meat from two year old bulls (mainly tenderness) appears acceptable and similar to that from intensively reared young bulls (Touraille, 1981).

This type of production is very efficient and is developing rapidly in some grassland regions producing beef, such as the Charolais or Aubrac areas (Lherm and Liénard, 1983).

Late maturing breeds, with high muscular growth potential, such as Charolais and Limousin, produce high carcass weights in steers as well as in bulls (Table 4). Early maturing breeds, such as Friesian, reared as bulls attain lower but adequate carcass weight without too much fat (Table 4). Unfortunately male behaviour problems occur with Friesian bulls grazing on pasture which limits their use. As steers, 2 year old Friesians produced fatty carcasses weighing only about 320 kg. Production of good carcasses from the Friesian breed is more suitable with autumn born cattle, slaughtered at 27-29 months of age, after an indoor fattening period.

Charolais cross-bred or dual purpose breeds such as Normand are well adapted to 2 year old bull and steer production (Table 4). Depending on their time of birth, they can produce 24 months old or 28 months old steers, mainly on grazed or conserved grass (Mourier, 1981).

It may be possible to further increase the part played by grass in beef production to reach the same proportion as in traditional systems, but with better performances. If the same feeding and management system

TABLE 3   Influence of level of feeding during the first winter on 2
year old beef production (Normand steers castrated at one year of age)

Level of feeding during first winter	High	Moderate	Low
n	24	24	24
First winter between 10 and 13 months - 111 d			
Initial weight (kg)	337	337	337
Average daily gain (g/d)	1043	807	640
Feed units/day	6.63	4.69	3.90
Feed efficiency (gain)	157	172	164
Grazing period between 14 and 20 months - 181 d			
Initial weight (kg)	471	440	419
Average daily gain (g/d)	613	664	751
Intensity of compensation	-	0.39	0.69
Fattening period between 21 and 24 months			
Initial weight (kg)	575	559	564
Average daily gain (g/d)	772	879	960
Duration (d)	70	79	72
Final weight (kg)	629	629	633
Feed units/day	7.48	7.45	7.84
Feed efficiency (gain)	103	118	122
Hot carcass weight (kg)	358	357	353
Carcass fat content (%)	18.8	17.9	17.6

(D. Micol, unpublished)

applied for 2 year old beef production is applied until 20 months of age,
it may be possible to extend production to 30-33 months.   Steers kept in
winter at low or moderate growth rate reach 550-600 kg at the end of
winter, and can be fattened on pasture to produce heavy carcasses at 30
months (Table 5).   Late born calves or light animals may have to be
fattened indoors in the following winter for slaughter at 33 months.   Only
steers and heifers can be used in this type of production to satisfy meat
quality requirements.   Results vary also with sex and breed.

TABLE 4   Influence of breed and sex on 2 year old beef production
(steers castrated at one year of age)(D.Micol,unpublished)

	Charolais bulls	Charolais steers	Normand bulls	Normand steers	Friesian bulls	Friesian steers	Limousin bulls	Normand bulls
n	7	7	8	8	8	8	12	12
First winter between 9 and 13 months								
Initial weight (kg)	301	299	320	323	306	304	313	300
Duration (d)	120	120	120	120	120	120	142	142
Average daily gain (g/d)	993	993	1027	919	934	880	972	968
Grazing period between 14 and 20 months								
Initial weight (kg)	417	421	429	422	408	401	429	420
Duration (d)	176	176	176	176	176	176	180	180
Average daily gain (g/d)	743	669	837	662	593	461	789	944
Fattening period between 21 and 24-25 months								
Initial weight (kg)	594	576	623	577	550	515	590	612
Duration (d)	83	103	65	68	60	64	91	91
Average daily gain (g/d)	1595	1149	1559	1160	1204	1243	1561	1418
Final weight (kg)	727	695	724	655	622	595	732	741
Feed units/day	8.37	8.02	9.75	8.67	8.96	8.64	9.95	10.58
Feed efficiency (g/FU)	190	143	160	134	134	144	157	134
Hot carcass weight (kg)	448	406	410	369	347	324	456	431
Carcass fat content (p 100)	12.0	16.4	14.3	18.8	15.4	19.7	15.8	18.0

(D Micol, unpublished data)

To obtain similar carcass weights with heifers as with 2 year old steers it is necessary to finish heifers at 28-30 months on pasture (Table 5). It may be possible to increase the carcass weight of heifers if they are fattened indoors between 30 and 35 months, with or without early calving before fattening. Some differences appear also between breeds with this system of production. For example, Limousin cattle always have lower growth rates than Normand cattle on pasture but the same growth rate and higher feed efficiency in indoor feeding, particularly on high energy diets (Tables 4 and 5). Thus, some breeds are better adapted to systems of production based on heavy and older animals, making maximal use of grassland.

CONCLUSION

Semi-intensive systems combined with efficient grazing management can achieve large improvements in grassland use for beef production in the

TABLE 5   Production of 30 month old beef cattle from steers and
heifers fattened on grass (steers castrated at one year of age)

	Limousin steers	Normand steers	Limousin heifers
n	12	12	12
First winter between 9 and 13 months			
Initial weight (kg)	318	297	292
Duration (d)	142	143	141
Average daily gain (g/d)	881	930	504
Grazing period between 14 and 20 months			
Initial weight (kg)	421	408	341
Duration (d)	168	168	166
Average daily gain (g/d)	678	848	693
Second winter between 21-25 months			
Initial weight (kg)	550	568	457
Duration (d)	117	117	117
Average daily gain (g/d)	415	360	410
Fattening period on grass between 26-30 months			
Initial weight (kg)	590	599	499
Duration (d)	122	114	120
Average daily gain (g/d)	729	938	705
Final weight (kg)	679	706	584
Hot carcass weight (kg)	409	391	341
Carcass fat content (%)	14.3	18.7	19.6

(D. Micol, 1982)

future. They are consistent with a reduction in cost of production due to
increased utilisation of grazed grass which remains the cheaper feed. They
also allow an increase in meat production per head of cattle and per
hectare, which will be more and more necessary in the future since the
number of dairy cows will decrease as will meat production capacity of
dairy breeds. This trend requires suitable animals with a large food

intake capacity for forages and grazed herbage and high muscle growth potential. Production of 2 year old bulls or heavy steers and heifers from continental beef breeds or crosses is in accordance with these objectives.

The majority of calves will come however from dairy herds, more and more from Holstein type, and it is necessary to define clearly their best utilisation, in particular through semi-intensive systems on grassland.

Moreover, these systems may be further improved as knowledge about them is increased and by the utilisation of additional technical parameters such as anabolic agents, feed additives and low cost winter feeding with by-products.

REFERENCES

Béranger, C. et Petit, M. 1971. Production de jeunes bovins de boucherie à partir d'herbe in "La Production de Viande par les jeunes bovins". Editions SEI-CNRA Versailles No **46**, 279-292.

Béranger, C. 1977. Grazing management for beef production. Proceedings of international meeting on animal production from temperate grassland. Dublin, June 1977. An Foras Taluntais, 126-130.

Faucon, A. 1981. Races bovines et production de viande. La Production Laitière Francaise I.N.R.A. Publ., 1981, 321-339.

G.E.B. 1982. La production de boeufs et de génisses de boucheries supplémenté à: Situation de marché des productions bovines No 92 I.T.E.B. - Group Economie Bovine - September 1982.

Le Du, J. 1980. Le paturage continu: l'expérience anglaise. Fourrages No 82, Juin 1980 31-43.

Lherm, M. et Liénard, 1983. Evolution récente des systèmes de production en troupeaux allaitants Charolais des zones herbagères. Bull. Tech. C.R.Z.V. Theix, I.N.R.A. (51) 63-83.

Micol, D. 1982. Production de boeufs et de génisses. Les principaux types de production de viande en race bovine Limousine. Bull. Tech. C.R.Z.V. Theix I.N.R.A. 1982 (48) 71-81.

Mourier, C. 1981. Comment produire des boeufs Normands pour l'abattage à 28-29 mois? Annuel pour l'éleveur bovin 1981 - I.T.E.B. 149 rue de Bercy, 75595 Paris Cedex 12;107-115.

Pousset. 1982. Evolution récente des productions fourragères en France et de leur intensification. Fourrages No 73, Mars 1978, 3-30. Actualisation 1981 - Communication personnelle.

Touraille, C. 1981. Influence du sexe et de l'âge de l'abattage sur les qualités organoleptiques des viandes de bovins limousins abattus entre 16 et 33 mois. Les principaux types de production de viande en race limousine. Bull. Tech. C.R.Z.V. Theix I.N.R.A. 1982 (48) 83-89.

SUMMER GRAZING AND WINTER FEEDING STUDIES WITH SUCKLER COWS

M.J. Drennan

The Agricultural Institute, Grange, Dunsany, Co. Meath, Ireland

ABSTRACT

Stocking rates of 2.47 (low), 3.71 (medium) and 4.94 (high) spring calving cows plus calves per ha were compared during three grazing seasons. Cows at the high stocking rate had lowest daily gains in all three years. Prior to early August, stocking rate had no effect on calf performance except in year 2 when those at the high stocking rate had lower daily gains. From early August until the end of the grazing season stocking rate significantly affected calf gains in all three years. Stocking rate had no effect on milk yield in year 1 but cows at the high stocking rate had reduced yields for most of year 2 and at the end of year 3. Regressions of calf daily gain from birth to the end of the season on milk yield of the cow were significant in all three years.

In two further experiments, beef cows were individually fed grass silage either to appetite (control) or 27 kg per head daily (restricted) during late pregnancy. All cows received silage to appetite during the first 42 (Experiment 1) or 49 days (experiment 2) of lactation and were subsequently grazed together at pasture. Plane of nutrition during late pregnancy affected cow liveweight changes. All cows lost weight during the first 6 to 7 weeks of lactation but recovered at pasture. Liveweight gains from 4 to 240 days post-calving in Experiment 1 for control and restricted cows were 33 and 84 kg respectively. The corresponding figures for the period 7 to 240 days post-calving in Experiment 2 were 70 and 95 kg. Plane of nutrition during late pregnancy did not influence the incidence of calving difficulties, feed intake during early lactation, milk production or cow fertility. Likewise, there was no effect of cow feeding level pre-calving on birth-weight or liveweight gain of calves in either experiment. Calf liveweight gains were significantly affected by milk yield of the dam.

INTRODUCTION

In suckled beef production the main saleable product is the weaned calf and thus calf growth rate is of prime importance. Although weight at culling is important, otherwise cow weights (or feeding levels) need only be sufficiently high to ensure no adverse effects on the cow (health, reproductive performance and longevity) or the calf (mortality and growth). As feed accounts for such a high proportion of total costs it is important to provide information on optimum feed requirements for the cow throughout the year and especially when feed costs are greatest. This will be influenced by the body condition (or weight) of the cow at the start of winter and the subsequent nutritional environment. The present studies were conducted to determine for a spring calving single suckler herd the effects of (1) stocking rate at pasture and (2) feeding level during winter pregnancy, on performance of cows and calves grazing good lowland pastures.

GRAZING STUDIES

Materials and Methods

During three grazing seasons, the effects of summer stocking rate on performance of spring calving suckler cows and their calves were studied (Drennan, 1971a and b). The treatments were as follows:

a. low stocking rate   - 2.47 cows (and calves) per ha
b. medium stocking rate - 3.71 cows (and calves) per ha
c. high stocking rate   - 4.94 cows (and calves) per ha

There were eight cows and calves in each treatment. The cows and calves were rotationally grazed around six paddocks of equal size. The cows were Hereford cross mated to a Hereford bull. First calving animals were used in year 1; the majority of the cows used in year 2 were also rearing their first calves and their second calves in year 3. Replacement Hereford cross calves were purchased where a calf died at parturition or shortly afterwards. Milk yield of the cows was estimated on eight, six and four occasions during years 1, 2 and 3 respectively using the calf suckling technique (Drennan, 1971a)

In year 1, the grazing season did not commence until 2 June but the grass was controlled earlier by a combination of grazing and cutting. Grazing commenced on 3 April and 11 April in years 2 and 3 respectively. Excess herbage was not removed but the pastures were topped when necessary. The grazing season ended each year when the animals at the high stocking rate were considered to be short of grass. About 1 month prior to grazing each year the pastures received 30 kg of phosphorus (P), 63 kg of potassium (K) and 58 kg of nitrogen (N) per ha. In addition, 29 kg of N per ha was applied in July of year 3.

RESULTS

Liveweight changes

The mean liveweights of the cows at the start were 355,368 and 405 kg in years 1,2 and 3 respectively. During the period from the start to early

August daily liveweight gains of the cows at the low stocking rate varied from 0.85 to 1.12 kg (Table 1). In this period, increasing the stocking rate from low to medium had no effect on cow gain during any of the three years.

TABLE 1   Effects of stocking rate at pasture on cow liveweight

| | Stocking rate | | | SE for treatment |
	Low	Medium	High	means
Liveweight change (kg/day)				
Early season				
Year 1 June 2 – Aug 4	0.86	0.92	0.76	±0.07
Year 2 April 3 – Aug 2	0.85[a]	0.78[a]	0.47[b]	±0.06
Year 3 April 11– Aug 1	1.12[a]	1.03[a]	0.77[b]	±0.07
Late season				
Year 1 Aug 4 – Oct 18	0.13[a]	0.00[a]	-0.19[b]	±0.06
Year 2 Aug 2 – Oct 4	0.13[a]	0.09[a]	-0.27[b]	±0.10
Year 3 Aug 1 – Sept 23	0.28[a]	-0.13[b]	-0.99[c]	±0.09
Entire season				
Year 1 June 2 – Oct 18	0.46[a]	0.42[a]	0.25[b]	±0.06
Year 2 April 3 – Oct 4	0.60[a]	0.54[a]	0.20[b]	±0.07
Year 3 April 11 – Sept 23	0.85[a]	0.65[b]	0.20[c]	±0.05

In this and subsequent tables values with different superscripts are significantly different(P<0.05)

Increasing the stocking rate from medium to high had no effect on gain in year 1 but reduced gain in years 2 (P<0.01) and 3 (P<0.05). From early August to the end of the grazing season increasing the stocking rate from low to medium reduced gain in year 3 only. Cows at the high stocking rate lost weight each year during this period and their performance was lower than that of cows at the medium stocking rate in all 3 years. Over the entire grazing season increasing the stocking rate from low to medium reduced cow performance in year 3 only. However, increasing the stocking rate from medium to high reduced cow weight gains in all three years.

Calf performance

Prior to early August the only significant effect of stocking rate on calf gain was in year 2 when calves at the high stocking rate had lower gains than calves at the low and medium rates (Table 2). From early August to the end of the grazing season calves at the low stocking rate continued to have daily gains in excess of 0.9 kg, but increase in stocking rate resulted in a significant reduction in calf gains in all 3 years.

TABLE 2   Effect of stocking rate at pasture on calf liveweight gains

	Stocking rate			SE for treatment means
	Low	Medium	High	
	Liveweight gain (kg/day)			
Early season				
Year 1 June 2 - Aug 4	0.95	0.94	0.92	±0.048
Year 2 April 3 - Aug 2	1.08[a]	1.03[a]	0.86[b]	±0.038
Year 3 April 11 - Aug 1	1.02	1.03	0.99	±0.055
Late season				
Year 1 Aug 4 - Oct 18	0.90[a]	0.74[b]	0.63[c]	±0.037
Year 2 Aug 2 - Oct 4	0.95[a]	0.73[b]	0.46[c]	±0.055
Year 3 Aug 1 - Sept 23	0.96[a]	0.76[b]	0.54[c]	±0.053
Entire season				
Year 1 June 2 - Oct 18	0.92[a]	0.83[ab]	0.76[b]	±0.034
Year 2 April 3 - Oct 4	1.04[a]	0.93[b]	0.72[c]	±0.037
Year 3 April 11 - Sept 23	1.00[a]	0.94[ab]	0.84[b]	±0.050

During the entire grazing season increasing the stocking rate from low to medium reduced calf daily liveweight gains in year 2 only. Likewise, increasing the stocking rate from medium to high reduced calf gains only in year 2. In all 3 years calf gains at the high stocking rate were less than at the low rate.

Milk yields

Estimated daily milk yields of the cows are shown in Table 3.   While the effects of stocking rate on yield followed the expected trends the only significant treatment differences were between the medium and high stocking on one occasion in year 2, the low and high stocking rates for most of year 2 and the final estimate in year 3.

TABLE 3 Mean milk yields of cows at different stocking rates

Age of Calves	Days	Date	Stocking rate			SE for treatment means
			Low	Medium	High	
			Milk yield (kg/day)			
Year 1	66	July 7	7.7	7.5	7.5	±0.60
	80	July 21	6.8	7.1	7.0	±0.55
	94	August 4	6.4	6.8	6.4	±0.52
	108	August 18	6.9	6.5	6.3	±0.54
	122	September 1	6.2	6.2	5.4	±0.47
	136	September 15	5.7	5.6	4.9	±0.45
	150	September 29	5.9	5.2	4.7	±0.51
	164	October 13	4.3	4.5	3.5	±0.40
Year 2	73	May 17	9.5^a	9.1^{ab}	6.8^b	±0.83
	101	June 14	8.6^a	7.7^{ab}	6.5^b	±0.57
	129	July 12	8.2^a	7.6^{ab}	6.2^b	±0.57
	150	August 2	7.5^a	7.4^a	5.2^b	±0.60
	171	August 23	7.8	7.1	5.2	±0.66
	199	September 20	5.4	5.3	4.1	±0.65
Year 3	97	June 6	8.6	9.6	8.8	±0.60
	125	July 4	8.9	10.2	8.8	±0.60
	153	August 1	8.5	9.0	7.1	±0.58
	195	September 12	8.2^a	7.6^{ab}	5.6^b	±0.69

Effect of milk yield on calf gain

A multiple regression equation of calf daily gain from birth to the end of the season, on milk yield of the cow, sex and age of calf, treatment and treatment by milk yield interaction was obtained. The factor showing greatest influence on calf growth was milk yield. For each kg increase in daily milk yield of the cow, daily liveweight gain of the calf from birth to the end of the season increased by 0.059 ($P<0.001$), 0.045 ($P<0.01$) and 0.057 kg, ($P<0.001$) in years 1, 2 and 3 respectively.

WINTER FEEDING STUDIES

Materials and methods

Two experiments were carried out using February/March calving Hereford cross cows which were individually fed during late pregnancy and for the first 42 (Experiment 1) or 49 days (Experiment 2) of lactation (Drennan and Bath, 1976 a & b). The following treatments were applied from housing in late November until calving:

1. Control - grass silage ad libitum
2. Restricted - grass silage restricted to 27 kg per head daily

After calving all cows were fed silage to appetite and then grazed together at pasture. The stocking rate at pasture was adjusted during the grazing season to ensure satisfactory animal performance throughout.

The cows used were from second to seventh parity and had been weaned a few weeks prior to the start of the experiments. The cows on Experiment 1 were mated with two Hereford bulls and those on Experiment 2 with two Friesian bulls. In each experiment, the cows were randomly allocated to the two treatments and in winter were tied in sawdust bedded cubicles. Calves were accommodated in spare cubicles close to their dams. Each cow reared her own calf only and the cow and calf remained together until the end of the grazing season.

Animal liveweights were recorded regularly throughout each experiment. Estimates of the cows' milk yields were obtained on 9 (Experiment 1) and 5 (Experiment 2) occasions by the calf suckling technique.

RESULTS
Cow liveweight changes

Mean liveweights and weight changes of the cows are shown in Table 4.

Reflecting the liveweight changes recorded during pregnancy, the control and restricted cows will be referred to as on high and medium planes of nutrition in Experiment 1 and as on medium and low planes in Experiment 2.

TABLE 4 Cow liveweights and weight changes in Experiments 1 and 2(kg)

| | Experiment 1 Plane of nutrition | | | Experiment 2 Plane of nutrition | | |
	High	Medium	F-test	Medium	Low	F-test
No. cows	12	11		13	16	
Initial wt	506±15	509±19	NS	500±18	502±16	NS
Wt 4 or 7 days post-calving	508±13	458±13	*	438±14	402±13	NS
Start to calving(days)	103±5	98±5	NS	79±4	77±3	NS
Wt change (kg/day)	0.02±0.07	-0.53±0.06	***	-0.74±0.08	-1.20±0.07	***
Wt changes						
4 or 7 to 60 days post-calving	-16±5	3±5	*	-9±3	-2±3	NS
4 or 7 to 120 days post-calving	18±7	54±7	**	38±5	59±5	*
4 or 7 to 240 days post-calving	33±9	84±9	***	70±6	95±6	**
Initial wt to 240 days post-calving	36±10	27±9	NS	8±5	-5±5	NS

Cow liveweights were over 500 kg at the start of both experiments. The average duration of the differential feeding period was 100 and 78 days in Experiments 1 and 2 respectively. In Experiment 1, control cows gained 2 kg liveweight from the start to 4 days post-calving whereas restricted cows lost 51 kg. The corresponding weight losses from the start to 7 days post-calving in Experiment 2 were 62 and 100 kg.

In both experiments, cows lost weight during the first 6 to 7 weeks of lactation but recovered at pasture. In both experiments, cows fed at a restricted level during late pregnancy gained significantly more liveweight during the subsequent grazing season. There was no significant difference between treatments in cow liveweight changes from the start of either experiment to 240 days post-calving.

Feed intakes

During late pregnancy in Experiment 1, high and medium plane animals consumed 8.5 and 5.1 kg of silage dry matter daily respectively (Table 5).

TABLE 5 Silage DM and metabolisable energy intakes in Experiments 1 & 2

Intake per day	EXPERIMENT 1 Plane of nutrition		EXPERIMENT 2 Plane of nutrition	
	High	Medium	High	Low
Silage DM (kg)				
Pregnancy	8.5	5.1	6.5	4.6
Lactation	8.7	8.8	7.1	7.0
ME (MJ)				
Pregnancy	77.4	46.4	53.6	38.1
Lactation	79.3	80.3	58.5	57.7

The corresponding figures for medium and low plane cows in Experiment 2 were 6.5 and 4.6 kg. There was no decline in silage intake with advancing pregnancy in either experiment. Plane of nutrition during late pregnancy had no significant effect on silage intakes during early lactation in either experiment although actual intakes in Experiment 2 were 8% higher in early lactation than in late pregnancy (unrestricted cows). Estimated daily metabolisable energy (ME) intakes during late pregnancy in Experiment 1 were 77.4 and 46.4 MJ for high and medium plane animals respectively. The corresponding figures for Experiment 2 were 53.6 and 38.1 MJ for medium and low plane cows respectively. The figure proposed (National Academy of Sciences, 1976) for a 500 kg beef cow during the last third of pregnancy is 68.6 MJ of ME. During early lactation daily ME intakes were about 79.9 and 58.2 MJ in Experiments 1 and 2 respectively. The proposed figure (NAS, 1976) for a 400 kg cow varies from 71 to 93 MJ depending on milking ability.

Calf birth weights, weight gains and calving difficulties

Plane of nutrition during late pregnancy had no significant effect on calf birth weights or growth rates in either experiment (Table 6). Likewise there was no effect of treatment on the incidence of difficult calvings in either study.

Milk production of cows

Plane of nutrition during late pregnancy had no significant effect on subsequent milk production in either experiment.

TABLE 6   Calf birth weights and weight gains in Experiments 1 & 2 (kg)

	EXPERIMENT 1 Plane of nutrition		F test	EXPERIMENT 2 Plane of nutrition		F test
	High	Medium		Medium	Low	
Birth weight	35.4±1.6	34.1±1.5	NS	37.4±0.9	37.3±0.8	NS
Gain birth to 60 days	39±2.1	44±2.2	NS	39±2.1	35±1.9	NS
Gain 60 to 120 days	58±2.3	62±2.4	NS	61±2.1	62±1.9	NS
Gain 120 to 180 days	57±1.9	58±1.9	NS	66±2.1	66±1.9	NS

Cow fertility

In Experiment 2 the number of days (± SE of treatment means) to fertile service for medium and low plane animals was 84.9 (±4.1) and 83.4 (±3.5) respectively.

Effect of milk yield on calf performance

The regression of calf gain from birth to weaning on average daily milk yield of the dam was obtained having adjusted for sex of calf. In Experiment 1, a 1 kg increase in daily milk yield resulted in 5.2 kg increase (P 0.05) in liveweight gain from birth to 180 days of age. In Experiment 2, a 1 kg increase in milk yield resulted in a 6.8 kg increase in calf gain from birth to 240 days.

DISCUSSION

In the grazing studies, increasing the stocking rate from 2.47 (low) to 3.71 (medium) cows plus calves per ha had no effect on cow or calf performance prior to August in any of the three years. A further increase from medium to high (4.94 cows plus calves per ha) reduced both cow milk yield and calf growth rate in year 2 only but cow liveweight gain was reduced in years 2 and 3. This indicates that stocking rates in the region of 3.71 to 4.94 cows plus calves per ha can be readily attained early in the grazing season. From early August to the end of the grazing season calves at the low stocking rate continued to have daily gains of over 0.9 kg. However, each successive increase in stocking rate resulted in a significant decrease in calf performance each year. In general, during this period cow liveweight changes and milk yield data followed a similar trend to the calves but differences were not always significant. These results show that in order to obtain high production per animal and per hectare the stocking rate must be adjusted downwards later in the season, in agreement with the findings of Conway (1968) with steers. Baker, Barker and Le Du (1982) also compared stocking rates of 4.12 (high) and 2.06 or 2.74 (low) spring calving cows and calves per ha over a four year period at the Grassland Research Institute, where rainfall is lower than in our own studies.Cows at the low stocking rate gained more weight than those at high stocking rates and in general gave more milk. Calf growth rates were also higher at low stocking rates in Experiments 1, 3 and 4 but not in Experiment 2. These workers concluded that the optimum stocking rate had probably been exceeded in these studies. They suggested that under their conditions for swards receiving 50 kg N per ha every 28 days four cows and calves per ha until June reducing to 2.75 or lower later in the season would be appropriate. Obviously the optimum figure will depend on factors such as soil and climatic conditions, fertiliser usage and date of commencing and ending the grazing season.

In the first winter feeding experiment, total liveweight losses in winter (pregnancy plus early lactation) of 27 and 78 kg were recorded for cows fed silage to appetite or restricted to 27 kg of silage daily during late pregnancy. The corresponding figures for Experiment 2 were 84 and 116 kg. These differences in winter liveweight losses of 51 and 32 kg in Experiments 1 and 2 respectively were offset by higher gains during the subsequent grazing season by previously restricted animals. During the grazing period cows previously restricted gained 44 and 21 kg more liveweight than their counterparts in Experiments 1 and 2 respectively. Jordan, Lister and Rowlands (1968a and b) using cows similar to those used in the present studies,have shown that with winter weight losses of up to 100 kg (20% of body weight) cow liveweights at the end of the grazing season were only slightly less than those recorded 12 months earlier. In that study losses of 60 to 70 kg in winter were completely recovered at weaning when compared with their counterparts fed a high plane of nutrition in winter, and yearly weight gains were about 18 kg.

In the present studies there was no effect of pre-calving level of nutrition on milk yield of the cows, calf birth weight or growth rates. In the study by Jordan et al with cows in good body condition initially, weight losses of about 0.1 kg liveweight daily during the last 120 days of pregnancy did not affect calf birth weights or subsequent calf growth rate. Russel, Peart, Eadie, MacDonald and White (1979) compared energy intakes ranging from 30 to 78 MJ ME daily during the last 84 days of pregnancy. Although there were treatment effects on calf birth weights there were no measurable effects on milk production or calf growth. Baker, Le Du and Barker (1982) and Hodgson, Peart, Russel, Whitelaw and MacDonald (1980) again showed the ability of animals to recover at pasture following severe energy restriction mainly during early lactation. In the latter studies there were minimal overall effects of restriction on total milk or final cow or calf weights. However, studies by Hight (1966, 1968a and b) in New Zealand have shown that severe energy restriction of light cows during winter pregnancy will depress subsequent calf performance.

In support of numerous other studies the present data show that cow milk is an important determinant of calf growth. The reason for the greater effect of milk production on weaning weight in the grazing studies was probably due to an overall lower average milk yield (about 7 kg daily) from these younger cows than those used in the winter feeding studies (8-9 kg of milk daily). In general, data in the literature support the view that the response to milk declines as the overall level of production increases.

CONCLUSIONS

Depending on climatic conditions, soil type and fertiliser usage, stocking rates of up to 4.5 spring calving cows plus calves per ha can be applied during the early part of the grazing season. However to maintain animal performance at a high level subsequently would involve a major reduction of the stocking rate. In practice this can be achieved by adjusting the overall stocking rate to about 2 cows and calves per ha, cutting about half the area twice for silage during the early season and grazing the entire area from August onwards. Under these conditions mature cows would be in good body condition at the start of winter and liveweight losses of 75 kg before calving could be tolerated without ill-effects on the cow or calf.

REFERENCES
Baker, R.D., Le Du, Y.L.P. and Barker, J.M. 1982. The influence of winter nutrition, grazing system and stocking rate on the performance of spring calving Hereford cross Friesian cows and their calves. 1. Winter nutrition. Anim. Prod. **34** 213-224
Baker, R.D., Barker, J.M. and Le Du, Y.L.P. 1982. The influence of winter nutrition, grazing system and stocking rate on the performance of spring calving Hereford cross Friesian cows and their calves. 2. Grazing system and stocking rate. Anim. Prod. **34** 225-237

Conway, A. 1968. Grazing management in relation to beef production. IV. Effect of seasonal variation in the stocking rate of beef cattle on animal production and on sward composition. Ir. J. agric. Res. **7** 93-104

Drennan,M.J. 1971a. Single-suckled beef production. 1. Influence of stocking rate during the grazing season. creep grazing of the calf and double-suckling on liveweight change and milk production of the cows. Ir. J. agric. Res. **10** 287-295

Drennan,M.J. 1971b. Single-suckled beef production. 2. Influence of stocking rate during the grazing season, creep grazing of the calf and double-suckling on calf performance. Ir. J. agric. Res. **10** 297-305

Drennan,M.J.and Bath, I.H. 1976a. Single-suckled beef production. 3. Effect of plane of nutrition during late pregnancy on cow performance. Ir. J. agric. Res. **15** 169-176

Drennan,M.J.and Bath, I.H. 1976b. Single-suckled beef production. 4. Effect of plane of nutrition during late pregnancy on subsequent calf performance. Ir. J. agric. Res. **15** 169-176

Hight,G.K. 1966. The effects of under nutrition in late pregnancy on beef cattle production. N.Z. J. Agric. Res. **9** 479-490

Hight,G.K. 1968a. Plane of nutrition effects in late pregnancy and during lactation on beef cows and their calves to weaning. N.Z. J.Agric.Res. **11** 71-84

Hight, G.K. 1968b. A comparison of the effects of three nutritional levels in late pregnancy on beef cows and their calves. N.Z. J. Agric. Res. **11** 477-486

Hodgson, J.,Peart, J.N. Russel,A.J.F., Whitelaw, A. and MacDonald, A.J. 1980. The influence of nutrition in early lactation on the performance of spring-calving suckler cows and their calves. Anim. Prod. **30** 315-325

Jordan, W.A., Lister, E.E. and Rowlands,G.J.1968a. Effect of plane of nutrition on wintering pregnant beef cows. Can. J. Anim. Sci. **48** 145-154

Jordan, W.A., Lister,E.E. and Rowlands, G.J. 1968b. Effect of varying planes of winter nutrition of beef cows on calf performance to weaning. Can. J. Anim. Sci. **48** 155-161

National Academy of Sciences,Nutrient requirement of beef cattle. Washington,DC.1976.

Russel,A.J.F., Peart, J.N., Eadie,J.,MacDonald,A.J. and White,I.R. 1979.The effect of energy intake during late pregnancy on the production from two genotypes of suckler cow. Anim. Prod. **28** 309-327

SOME EFFECTS OF CHANGES IN COW LIVEWEIGHT IN THE AUTUMN CALVING
SUCKLER HERD

D.M.B. Chestnutt

Agricultural Research Institute, Hillsborough, Co. Down, N. Ireland.

ABSTRACT

Autumn-calving suckler cows can make large gains at grass when feed cost is low, and the resulting body reserves can be used to reduce winter feed costs. Cows which gained 138 kg at grass between mid-April and the end of August and lost 100 kg over the winter, produced calves which were 28 kg lighter in June than cows which gained 25 kg between April and August and a further 13 kg over the winter. However, because of higher winter feed costs in the latter system, economic considerations would favour the former. The type of ration fed to cows in negative energy balance appeared to influence the efficiency with which body reserves were used. Calves gained 1.18 kg/d where cows lost 0.52 kg/d on a ration of silage plus 0.75 kg/d fish meal, compared with a gain of 0.95 kg/d where cows lost 0.59 kg/d on a ration of silage alone.

INTRODUCTION

When suckler cows calve near the end of the grazing season the late lactation and dry period correspond with the time when there may be an ample supply of grass which could be used to increase body reserves. These can then be used to remedy an imposed negative energy balance in the cow over the winter when food is generally more expensive. This involves the conversion of food energy to body reserves, body reserves to milk and milk to weight gain in the calf, each process being associated with some degree of energy loss. However, the efficiency of conversion of body reserves to milk is high (Moe and Flatt, 1969) and it seems that where the difference between costs of summer grazing and of winter feeding is high there could be an economic benefit from the use of weight gained during the grazing season to produce milk in the winter period.

At the Agricultural Research Institute of Northern Ireland a herd of Aberdeen Angus x British Friesian cows is intensively managed on lowland pasture. This herd grazes for approximately six months from mid-April to mid-October and the mean calving date is around 20 September. Cows are housed over winter when the main feed is grass silage, with concentrate offered to cows as necessary. Over the past few years factors affecting the liveweight of cows and the effect of change in cow liveweight on calf performance have been examined.

Effect of weaning date

Comparisons have been made between weaning just before cows are turned out to pasture in early April and weaning in early July (Chestnutt, 1980). In agreement with other studies (Powell, 1975 and Lowman, Donaldson and Edwards, 1978) calves gained more weight when weaning date was deferred. Calves weaned in July were 29 kg heavier than those weaned earlier but at this stage their mothers were 33 kg lighter than the mothers of earlier-weaned calves. When kept under uniform conditions until the end of August the difference in calf weight in favour of late weaning was 22 kg while their mothers were 22 kg lighter than where weaning took place at turn out to pasture. There would thus seem to be a useful advantage in weaning after a period of suckling at pasture provided cow liveweight can be restored before calving in September. When good-quality pasture was available to calves, suckled milk yield tended to fall fairly rapidly from a peak of 8 kg/d after turnout to grass to about 3 kg/d in late June. In terms of increased calf liveweight the benefit to be gained from suckling during June is small and the optimum weaning date is probably early in June. Cows weaned in June and calved in September have ample opportunity to build up body reserves at pasture for use in reducing winter feed requirements.

Liveweight gain of cows at grass

In Northern Ireland summer temperatures of 15-20°C with 300 to 400 millimetres of rainfall distributed fairly uniformly over the summer months form a good basis for grass production. With an input of 400 kg nitrogen/ha cut yields of 13,000 kg dry matter/ha are commonly achieved. Under these circumstances autumn-calving cows will generally gain weight while suckling calves after turnout to pasture in early April. Over a number of years an average weight gain of 0.43 kg/d was recorded in cows between early April and early July with a stocking rate of 5 cows and their calves per hectare. After weaning the capacity for weight increase will obviously be greater.

Experimental

In an experiment over three years (1977-1981) 18 Aberdeen Angus x British Friesian cows were weaned in early April each year and subjected to three different stocking rates until the end of August to obtain three levels of body reserve for use during the following winter. The cows were allocated to areas in the ratio of 100 (H) to 80 (M) to 75 (L) in the first year and in the second and third years this ratio was changed to 100 (H) to 76 (M) to 67 (L). The effect on animal performance is shown in Table 1.

Grazing was on a rotational basis in a five week grazing cycle on an area greater than that required to sustain the experimental animals. Any residual grass after 5 weeks was grazed by other cattle similar to those on experiment. The stocking rate in Table 1 is based on the mean area utilised during each grazing cycle. Daily gains approaching 1 kg from the beginning of April resulted in cows on the H treatment being 114 kg heavier than those on the L treatment by the end of August. Cows from all

TABLE 1   Effect of area per cow on liveweight gain between early April and late August (average of 3 years)

Area per cow	High (H)	Medium (M)	Low (L)	SE
Relative mean pasture area	100	77.3	69.7	-
Mean stocking rate (cows/ha)	10.7	13.9	15.7	-
Liveweight gain (kg/d)	0.93	0.47	0.1	0.109

treatments were then grazed as a single group through the calving period with adequate pasture until 20 October when they were housed. During the calving period there was some evidence of compensation with mean losses of 38, 29 and 27 kg on H, M and L treatments respectively so that cows on the H treatment had gained 103 kg more at the start of the winter feeding period than those on the L treatment.

At all three levels of stocking grass utilisation was high. During periods of wet weather there was some poaching but this did not necessitate removal of animals from pasture at any stage. In the third year pasture production and utilisation on H and L treatments between 21 May and 3 September was measured by cutting sample areas to ground level before and after a 2-day grazing period in each week. No account was taken of growth during this grazing period. Results are summarised in Table 2.

TABLE 2   Mean offered and residual yield, intake and herbage production between 21 May and 3 September 1979.

Area per cow	High (H)	Low (L)	SE
Pasture on offer (kg DM/ha)	3973	3403	113.6
Post grazing residue (kg DM/ha)	1156	1008	42.3
Daily intake (kg DM/cow)	6.80	3.86	0.228
Herbage production (kg/ha)	8727	7651	

The fact that grazing residue differed little between treatments probably indicates that this is approaching the minimum pasture residue possible for animals of this type.   Nevertheless it appears that the difference in residue or the trampling effect of the extra density of stock on the L treatment reduced herbage production on this treatment.   Such a reduction at higher stocking rate agrees with the findings of McFeely, Butler and Gleeson (1977).

Based on liveweight and liveweight change of cows it was calculated that mean output of Utilized Metabolisable Energy ME (UME) was 112, 116 and 99 GJ/ha for H, M and L treatments respectively from the start of grazing until the end of August.   Thus it would appear that the stocking rate required for maximum UME output was within the range used.   In keeping with the results of the cutting experiment (Table 2) a substantial reduction in UME was evident at the highest stocking rate.

The H treatment which involved higher intake of energy in late pregnancy might have been expected to increase calf birth weight and hence dystokia (Tudor, 1972).   There was no evidence of this with little difference between birthweights on H and L treatments.   The fact that extra energy on the H treatment was supplied in the form of forage rather than concentrate may have been important in this respect (Lowman et al,1978)

Weight change over winter

Cows in the experiments described above were subjected to different winter feeding levels designed to cause a loss of the extra weight gained on H and M treatments during the grazing season.   Cows on the L treatment were fed at a level designed to maintain liveweight throughout the winter. The winter ration consisted mainly of grass silage containing on average 182 g/kg dry matter with 23.4 g/kg nitrogen, 392 g/kg MAD fibre and 90 g/kg ash in the dry matter. The mean D value was 63.2 and all silages were well preserved with a mean pH of 4.1. These silages were also offered ad libitum to calves in a separate creep area. A concentrate supplement consisting of ground barley with added minerals and vitamins and having 851 g/kg dry matter with 16 g/kg nitrogen, 60 g/kg crude fibre, 49 g/kg ash in the dry matter was offered in the M and L treatments.

Winter feeding on the H treatment consisted of silage, restricted as necessary to achieve the desired loss of liveweight. On the L treatment silage was offered ad libitum to a 10% residue (about 5 kg) and concentrate supplementation was adjusted to achieve a stable liveweight while on the M treatment silage was restricted by accepting a lower residue (about 1 kg) and concentrate level was adjusted to achieve the desired weight loss. The effect of silage and concentrate intake on the daily weight loss over winter is shown in Table 3.

TABLE 3   Intake of silage and concentrate, and weight change in cows between 3 November and 5 April (kg/d)

Level of summer gain	High (H)	Medium (M)	Low (L)	SE
Silage DM intake	7.53	8.83	9.78	0.320
Concentrate DM intake	0	0.68	1.39	0.083
Weight change	−0.65	−0.35	0.08	0.097

Using ME values derived from D values (0.15 x D) for silages and 13 MJ/kg for concentrate DM, mean total ME intake values for the winter period were 11.0 GJ, 13.3 GJ and 17.3 GJ for H, M and L treatments respectively. Using a value of 38 MJ ME/kg weight loss in the cow, the energy available for maintenance and milk production can be calculated as 14.8, 16.4 and 16.7 GJ on H, M and L treatments respectively.

The effect of treatment on the intake and performance of calves during the winter period is given in Table 4.

TABLE 4   Effect of treatments on the intake and performance of calves (kg/d)

Level of summer gain	High (H)	Medium (M)	Low (L)	SE
Suckled milk yield	7.08	8.51	9.76	0.251
Silage DM intake	1.54	1.38	1.44	0.066
Liveweight gain	0.85	1.02	1.09	0.028

Suckled milk yield was significantly greater when cows were fed to maintain weight (L) than where they were kept in negative energy balance and expected to mobilise body reserves to provide part of the energy for milk production (H and M). Silage intake of calves, which increased from 0.27 kg/d in mid-November to 2.78 kg/d in early April, was not significantly affected by milk yield. Liveweight gain in calves reflected the milk yield and calves of cows on the H treatment were 37 kg lighter than those cows on the L treatment by the end of the winter.

Assuming a requirement of 5.2 MJ ME/kg milk produced and a maintenance requirement of 48 MJ/d for a 500 kg cow the total utilised ME over the winter period can be calculated as 12.5, 13.8 and 14.9 GJ for H, M and L treatments respectively. The fact that these are lower than the calculated ME available may be related to the conversion values used or perhaps to the fact that suckled milk yield may have been underestimated (Chestnutt, 1982).

It is evident that cows on the low plane of nutrition over the winter period had less energy available for production and this was reflected in lower levels of utilised energy. Despite higher levels of body reserves on the H treatment the reduction in energy intake necessary to achieve mobilisation of this reserve was greater than the energy yield from the reserve. This could be due to inadequate mobilisation of reserves or to inefficient utilisation of mobilised reserve.

The 37 kg weight advantage of calves on the L treatment at weaning in early April was reduced to 28 kg when the calves grazed as a single group until early June. This extra 28 kg liveweight associated with the L treatment was obtained at the expense of 250 kg concentrate and approximately 2 tonnes of silage (the area required to provide for the extra gain during the grazing season on the H treatment was roughly equal to the area required to make the extra silage consumed on the L treatment). In economic terms the cost of the extra feeding required is too high and better returns would be achieved by allowing cows to deposit substantial body reserves during the grazing season and to use these to reduce the cost of the winter diet. However, calves have been shown to have a potential to gain at rates in excess of 1 kg daily during the winter and obviously gains of this order would be more acceptable if they could be achieved economically.

Effect of winter ration given to suckler cows in negative energy balance

It has been shown by Robinson, Frazer, Gill and McHattie (1974) with ewes and by Ørskov, Grubb and Kay (1977) with cows, that more dietary protein is necessary when animals are in negative energy balance. It was decided therefore to investigate the effect of protein level and source on the efficiency of use of body reserves by the suckling cow over winter. The first experiment in this series has been completed and the main findings are summarised below.

In this experiment the effect of fixed levels of barley meal and fish meal with silage offered to cows in negative energy balance over the winter period was compared with cows on silage alone and with cows on a diet of silage ad libitum with concentrate as necessary to maintain weight. A total of 32 Aberdeen Angus x British Friesian cows was divided into four uniform groups of eight. Three groups were managed at pasture to gain about 120 kg between weaning in early June and calving in September. Pasture availability was restricted with the fourth group so that over the same period liveweight gain was approximately 60 kg. From housing in mid-October until 23 December all cows were given silage ad libitum with concentrate as required to maintain the liveweight at housing. Insemination commenced on 20 November and continued until mid-January. The four treatments imposed between 23 December and 6 April consisted of:-

a. 0.75 kg white fish meal per day with silage restricted
    to achieve target weight loss of 100 kg.

b. 0.75 kg ground barley per day with silage restricted to
    achieve target loss of 100 kg.

c. Silage restricted to achieve target weight loss of 100 kg.

d. Cows which had been restricted in weight gain during the
    grazing season were offered silage ad libitum with barley
    adjusted as necessary to maintain liveweight through the winter.

Cows were rationed behind individual Calan-Broadbent doors and feeding levels were adjusted on the basis of twice weekly weighings with the object of achieving set target weights by 8 April. Results are given in Table 5.

Due to a technical problem with the animal balance liveweight loss during the winter was less than desired, averaging just over 0.5 kg/day in treatments A, B and C while in treatment D a liveweight gain of the order of 0.1 kg/day occurred. In keeping with earlier results liveweight loss achieved by reducing silage consumed (treatment C) was accompanied by a significant reduction in milk yield and in calf performance when compared with cows where liveweight was maintained (treatment D). Both milk yield and calf performance were improved when part of the nutrient intake of animals on negative balance was barley (treatment B). Where fish meal was included (treatment A) milk yield was equal to that obtained with treatment D and the calf daily liveweight gain was significantly higher than where barley was used (treatment B)

TABLE 5   Effect of ration and weight loss of cows on suckled milk yield and calf performance (23 December-8 April)

Treatment	Weight loss (kg)	Feed consumption (kg DM/d) Silage	Concentrate	Milk yield (kg/d)	Calf LWG (kg/d)
A	55	5.71	0.68 (Fish)	8.8	1.18
B	51	6.82	0.64 (Barley)	7.4	1.00
C	63	7.10	0	6.5	0.95
D	-13	8.54	1.42 (Barley)	8.8	1.10
SE	6.3	0.403		0.45	0.044

Calculating energy available on the basis of 10.1 MJ ME per kg silage DM, 13.0 MJ ME/kg ground barley DM, 11.0 MJ ME/kg white fish meal DM and assuming additivity of concentrate and silage ME, total feed ME was 6.91 GJ, 8.19 GJ, 7.61 GJ and 11.11 GJ from December to April in treatments A, B, C and D respectively. This represents a mean 32% saving in energy intake over the experimental period where animals were fed to lose weight in the first three treatments, compared with treatment D.

Using values of 48 MJ/d for maintenance of a 500 kg cow and 5.2 MJ/kg milk produced, values for utilised ME were 9.68 GJ, 8.87 GJ, 8.43 GJ and 9.37 GJ for treatments A, B, C and D respectively. If we assume that the difference between feed energy and utilised energy was accounted for by use of body tissue, and use weight loss as a measure of that body tissue the energy values of weight loss were 50.4, 13.3 and 13.0 MJ ME per kg for treatments A, B and C respectively. While a value of 50.4 MJ/kg indicates the likelihood of some change in the water content of body tissue, it is obvious that energy available on treatment A was used much more efficiently than on treatments B and C. Subsequent weight changes of these cows under uniform conditions at pasture were similar on all three treatments. The most likely cause of increased efficiency of milk production where a protein source of low rumen degradability is used under conditions of negative energy balance would appear to be the more efficient utilization of body reserves. Ørskov, Reid and McDonald (1981) obtained a milk yield increase from dairy cows using fish meal as opposed to groundnut meal only where animals were drawing heavily on body reserves.

Thus, white fish meal allowed body reserves to be used over the winter without a reduction in energy available. The cost of fish meal is high in relation to barley meal and while there was a considerable saving in silage when fish meal was used (comparing treatments A and D) a greater area of grassland was necessary in order to achieve the extra liveweight at the time of housing on treatment A. It is hoped in future years to further investigate the effect of variations in the level of fish meal included in the diet and to evaluate other sources of protein of low degradability.

REFERENCES
Chestnutt, D.M.B. 1980. Effect of suckling frequency on milk yield of single-suckler cows. Record of Agricultural Research, Department of Agriculture, Northern Ireland, 28, 97.
Chestnutt, D.M.B. 1982. The effect of weaning date on the performance of autumn-calving, single-suckled cows. Animal Production 34: 71.
Lowman, B.G., Donaldson, E. and Edwards, R.A. 1978. The effect of time of weaning on the performance of suckled calves. Animal Production 26: 381.
McFeely, P.C., Butler, T.M. and Gleeson, P.A. 1977. Potential of Irish grassland for dairy production. Proceedings of the International Meeting on Animal Production from Temperate Grassland, Dublin, 1977. Ed. B. Gilsenan, p 5.
Moe, P.W. and Flatt, W.P. 1969. Use of body tissue reserves for milk production by the dairy cow. Journal of Dairy Science 52: 928.
Ørskov, E.R., Grubb, D.A. and Kay, R.N.B. 1977. Effect of postruminal glucose or protein supplementation on milk yield and composition in Friesian cows in early lactation and negative energy balance. British Journal of Nutrition 38: 397.
Powell, T.L. 1975. Winter feeding and date of weaning in the early autumn calving single suckler herd. Experimental Husbandry No 29, 61.
Robinson, J.J., Fraser, C., Gill, J.C. and McHattie, I. 1974. Effect of dietary crude protein concentration and time of weaning on milk production and body-weight change in the ewe. Animal Production 19: 331.
Tudor, G.D. 1972. The effect of pre- and post-natal nutrition on the growth of beef cattle. I. The effect of nutrition and parity of the dam on calf birth weight. Australian Journal of Agricultural Research 23: 389.

THE PERFORMANCE OF BEEF COWS AND THEIR CALVES AT PASTURE

I.A. Wright, J. Hodgson and A.J.F. Russel

Hill Farming Research Organisation, Bush Estate, Penicuik, Midlothian, EH26 0PY, United Kingdom

INTRODUCTION

Grazed grass can account for 60-80% of the annual nutrient intake in beef cow systems in Northern Europe and it is therefore important that the factors which influence the performance of beef cows and their calves at pasture are clearly understood. The effects on production of nutrition during both the grazing season and the preceding winter will be discussed.

The effect of winter nutrition on performance at pasture

Forty-eight Hereford x Friesian and Shorthorn x Galloway cows were fed hay to supply about 75% of the estimated maternal maintenance energy requirements for the last 12 weeks of pregnancy. From calving in February-March the cows were fed to supply the theoretical requirement for either 2.25 kg (L) or 9.0 kg (H) milk per day. At turn-out in mid-May the cows and calves were grazed as a single herd on a rotational grazing system with a daily herbage allowance of 50 g DM/kg total live weight of cows and calves. Full experimental details are given by Hodgson, Peart, Russel, Whitelaw and Macdonald (1980).

Results are given in Table 1 and Figure 1. During early lactation H cows gave more milk than L cows and consequently their calves grew faster and were heavier when turned out to grass. Treatment L cows lost more weight than those on Treatment H and were in lower body condition when turned out. All cows showed a considerable increase in milk yield at turn-out, the increase being greatest in the L cows. Throughout the grazing season the L cows consistently gave more milk than the H cows resulting in faster calf growth. Weight gains in the L cows were also higher. The higher milk yields and weight gains of the L cows appear to be due to greater herbage intake. It is possible that the higher intakes of the L cows were due to their lower body condition at turn-out rather than the lower level of winter feeding per se.

Sward conditions and animal performance

In a second experiment thirty-two cows (equal numbers of Hereford x

TABLE 1   The effect of winter feed level on performance at pasture

Feed level	L	H	s.e.
Winter			
Cow			
Milk yield (kg/day)	8.1	9.5	0.26
Weight loss (kg/day)	1.73	1.26	0.144
Condition score at turnout	2.2	2.4	0.14
Calf			
Live-weight gain (kg/day)	0.77	0.93	0.038
Weight at turnout (kg)	80	86	1.7
Summer			
Cow			
Milk yield (kg/day)	11.7	10.8	0.60
Live-weight gain (kg/day)	0.35	0.21	0.053
Condition score at weaning	2.9	2.8	0.13
Herbage intake (kg OM/day)	14.1	13.6	0.33
Calf			
Live-weight gain (kg/day)	1.17	1.14	0.024
Weaning weight (kg)	219	223	4.0

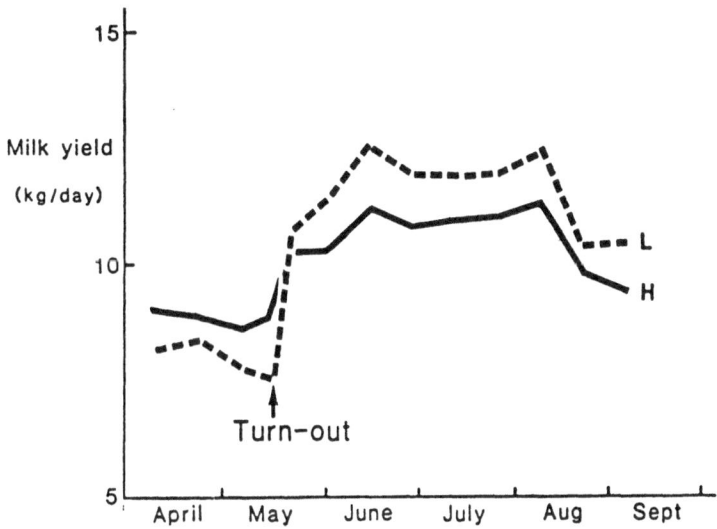

Fig. 1 Mean daily milk yield

Friesian and Shorthorn x Galloway) and their spring-born calves grazed perennial ryegrass swards maintained at minimal sward surface heights of 4-5 cm (S) and 8-10 cm (T). Sward height was measured by the use of a device developed by Bircham (1981). Cows were either maintained on treatment, or switched between treatments for three successive periods of 6 weeks. Actual herbage heights and masses are given in Table 2. The results

TABLE 2   Herbage height and mass

	Herbage height (cm)		Herbage mass (kg DM/ha)	
	S	T	S	T
Period 1	8.3	9.8	2100	2800
2	4.2	7.5	1500	2900
3	4.4	6.8	1600	3000

(Table 3) indicate that the height of the sward influenced cow live-weight gain and milk yield, with the higher gains, milk yields and calf growth rates occurring on the 8-10 cm sward. A higher stocking rate was required to maintain the lower of the two swards (Table 4) and despite lower individual calf performance,this resulted in a higher total calf gain per hectare.

TABLE 3   The effect of herbage height on animal performance

	Cow LWG (kg/day)			Milk yield (kg/day)			Calf LWG (kg/day)		
	S	T	se	S	T	se	S	T	se
Period 1	0.28	0.82	0.070	10.1	11.1	0.55	0.97	1.28	0.047
2	-0.78	0.42	0.089	9.4	11.0	0.49	0.88	1.29	0.064
3	0.17	-0.15	0.132	9.2	9.9	0.35	1.19	1.18	0.067
mean	-0.11	0.36		9.6	10.7		1.01	1.25	

TABLE 4   Stocking rates and calf gain per hectare

Herbage height	S	T
Stocking rate (cows/ha)		
May	5.0	3.5
September	2.5	2.0
Calf gain per ha (kg)	450	400

CONCLUSIONS

The performance of beef cows and their calves at pasture is influenced by both current and previous nutrition. Cows on a low plane of nutrition in early lactation on winter diets have a higher herbage intake at pasture, resulting in increased live-weight gain, milk yield and calf growth rate. Savings in winter feed can be made by letting cows draw on their body reserves and then allowing them to replenish these reserves at pasture when the provision of nutrients is relatively cheap. However, to take full advantage of this, grassland management must allow the provision of sufficient high quality herbage to allow cows to regain fully the weight and body condition lost during the winter. Although high summer stocking rates may lead to increased output of weaned calf per hectare, the resulting short swards may not allow cows to regain weight adequately.

REFERENCES

Bircham, J.S. 1981. Herbage growth and utilisation under continuous management. PhD thesis, University of Edinburgh.

Hodgson, J. Peart, J.N., Russel, A.J.F., Whitelaw, A. and Macdonald, A.J. 1980. The influence of nutrition in early lactation on the performance of spring-calving suckler cows and their calves. Anim. Prod. **30** 316-325.

GRASP - A GRASSLAND PLANNING PROGRAM FOR THE HP41C PROGRAMMABLE CALCULATOR

A.W. Spedding

Meat and Livestock Commission, PO Box 44, Queensway House, Bletchley,
Milton Keynes, MK2 2EF

ABSTRACT

The 'GRASP' program has been produced as an advisory aid for use on farms by MLC beef and sheep specialists. The program uses information about rainfall, soil type, grass species and proposed N fertiliser use to calculate potential stocking during each sixth of the grazing season. Potential is then used to calculate the grazing needs during each sixth of the season for the stock to be carried on the area concerned. Areas not needed for grazing are then available to be cut for silage. The total quantity of silage which should be made is shown. If this does not match the winter needs for silage, inputs can be adjusted until both grazing needs and silage needs are met.

Variations in stocking rate through the grazing season were recorded in 1982 on 333 farms. There was a wide range in the level of stocking, but differences in stocking pattern between different soil types and at different levels of rainfall were less than expected. Areas which were cut mainly for silage had higher levels of production early in the season than areas where grazing and conservation were integrated but thereafter production from silage areas was lower. Areas which were mainly grazed showed much more level stocking through the season than integrated areas.

It seems likely that the program will need to be modified to take more account of records of previous levels of stocking and of the balance of grazing and conservation.

INTRODUCTION

Results from the Meat and Livestock Commission beef recording scheme BEEFPLAN have shown a wide range in stocking rate in British beef enterprises. Table 1 shows the relationship between N fertiliser applied and stocking rate expressed as Livestock Units (LU) per ha.

(LU = average liveweight x 0.00215)

Table 1 shows a steady increase in stocking rate as N fertiliser increased. But since two thirds of the enterprises recorded used less than 200 kg N there is clearly further scope on many farms for increasing N fertiliser use. There was little evidence of reduced cattle performance even at the highest levels of stocking (Table 2)

The amount of N fertiliser applied was closely related to stocking rate up to about 3.0 LU per ha, but at higher stocking rates the relationship with N fertiliser was not so consistent. The results indicate that high stocking rates were being achieved on some farms without the highest level of N fertiliser use. Moreover, there was no evidence of a decline in daily gain at higher stocking rates to indicate that cattle

TABLE 1 N fertiliser and stocking rate - 1982 results

N fertiliser (kg/ha)	No of records	Stocking rate (LU/ha)
0 - 50	31	1.9
51-100	86	2.4
101-150	113	2.8
151-200	93	3.3
201-250	87	3.6
251-300	60	3.9
301-350	35	4.1
351+	26	4.5

TABLE 2 Relationship between stocking rate, N fertiliser and daily liveweight gain - 1982

Stocking rate (LU/ha)	No of records	N fertiliser (kg/ha)	Liveweight gain (kg/day)	(kg/ha)
1.0-1.5	3	98	0.6	233
1.5-2.0	13	91	0.7	381
2.0-2.5	30	126	0.7	470
2.5-3.0	51	146	0.8	626
3.0-3.5	44	201	0.8	695
3.5-4.0	37	203	0.7	747
4.0-4.5	27	216	0.8	862
4.5-5.0	16	200	0.7	855
5.0+	24	245	0.8	975

were overstocked.

Many factors influence grass growth; the amount and seasonality of rainfall, type of sward, soil type, level of N fertiliser, as well as the way the sward is managed for grazing or conservation. Many beef producers find the planning of stocking rates so difficult that they understock to ensure that there will always be sufficient grass. The GRASP program is used as part of a strategy for grazing management to encourage producers to increase stocking. The program gives priority to grazing requirements by first calculating the amount of grassland needed for each group of stock in each month of the grazing season. The amount and timing of silage to be cut from the area not needed for grazing is then calculated. This is checked by the MLC Beef Specialist to ensure that enough silage can be made for the winter needs of the unit. If insufficient silage is indicated, the effect on silage supply of an increase in N fertiliser can be calculated.

CALCULATION OF POTENTIAL STOCKING RATE

The program calculates potential stocking rate taking account of four factors, rainfall, soil type, level of N fertilizer and grass species:

1. Rainfall

Annual rainfall at the site is used to determine the average stocking rate in kg liveweight per hectare which would be possible at 150 kg of N fertiliser per hectare. The average stocking rate achieved by members of BEEFPLAN in 1981 has been used at 600-725 mm rainfall, and stocking rates at other levels of rainfall are derived from differences in herbage production due to annual rainfall shown in the ADAS/GRI GM20 trials,(Morrison et al,1980)

The average stocking rates, which are inputs for the program, are shown in Table 3.

TABLE 3 Average stocking rates in relation to annual rainfall

Annual rainfall (mm)	600	600-725	725-850	850
Average stocking rate (kg liveweight/ha)	1230	1360	1490	1620

If rooting depth is restricted by shallow soil or poor drainage or if altitude is greater than 250 metres the stocking rate entered into the program is reduced by one level (eg 1620 to 1490 kg)

2. Soil type

An adjustment is entered to allow for differences in average production due to soil type. Further factors are entered to calculate the stocking rate which should be possible in each sixth of the grazing season. These factors are shown in Table 4.

The adjustments for soil type are derived from the GM20 trials. The factors used to determine the availability of grass through the season have been derived from several sources and assume that lighter soils warm up more quickly than heavier soils, dry up more in mid-summer but produce more usable grass in the autumn.

TABLE 4   Effects of soil type on stock carrying capacity

	Sand & gravel	Sandy loam	Medium loam & silt	Clay loam	Heavy clay
			Multiplication factors		
Overall stocking capacity LU/ha	0.65	0.80	1.01	0.90	0.80
Stock carrying capacity as a proportion of the annual average					
First sixth of season	1.50	1.45	1.40	1.20	1.10
Second sixth " "	1.40	1.40	1.40	1.40	1.40
Third sixth " "	0.70	0.80	0.90	1.00	1.10
Fourth sixth " "	0.65	0.70	0.75	0.80	0.85
Fifth sixth " "	0.80	0.75	0.70	0.75	0.80
Sixth sixth " "	0.95	0.90	0.85	0.85	0.75

3.   N fertiliser

The amount of fertiliser nitrogen proposed for the whole grazing season is entered and the program then calculates further adjustment factors. The amount of fertiliser proposed may need to be adjusted for presence of clover in the sward and for organic manures applied to the grassland. Adjustment for clover is done only if more than 30 per cent of the sward is made up of clover (Table 5)

TABLE 5   Nitrogen contribution from clover

Applied nitrogen (kg/ha)	Nitrogen contribution from clover (kg/ha)
nil	150
100	90
200	30
> 250	nil

The program assumes a straight-line response in stocking rate to N up to 300 kg N per ha, starting from a base of 650 kg of liveweight stocked per hectare when no N fertiliser is applied (medium loam soil, 725-800 mm rainfall). Up to 300 kg N per ha this stocking rate is adjusted by a multiplication factor of 1.0035 kg liveweight for each kg per ha of N. Above 300 kg N per ha the adjustment is 1.0017 kg liveweight for each kg per ha of N.

4. Grass species

Production potential is adjusted by entering a factor of 0.90 if the swards are made up of predominantly fine-leaved rather than broad-leaved grasses. Grass species are likely to be a more important limitation at N levels in excess of 300 kg N per ha, but it is unlikely that such levels of fertiliser would be recommended on swards containing the less productive species.

CALCULATION OF GRAZING STOCK REQUIREMENTS

Once the potential stocking rate for each sixth of the grazing season has been calculated the program uses cattle weight at turnout to pasture, daily gain and stock numbers to calculate the total liveweight to be stocked in each sixth of the season. The potential stocking rate for each sixth is then used to calculate the number of grazing hectares needed in each sixth. Any land not required for grazing according to this calculation is assumed to be cut for silage. The potential stocking rate is used to calculate the liveweight which could be stocked on the conservation area and this is then converted to its equivalent as silage (250 g DM per kg) using the MLC livestock unit system.

AMENDING INPUTS

Inputs can be amended singly or together and the effect on grazing requirements shown so that if the first run does not give a satisfactory answer alternatives can be examined. Where drastic shortages seem likely, the effect of either increasing the grassland available or removing stock can be calculated. If available, the site information can be replaced by actual recorded stocking rates and fertiliser usage.

However accurately a grazing plan is drawn up, it needs to be flexible enough to cope with the vagaries of the weather. Producers are advised to adopt a grazing buffer which is used only if the main grazing area is insufficient. The buffer is usually about 20 per cent of the grazing area indicated by the GRASP program. If both the main grazing area and the buffer are used, animal performance should be sustained with supplementary concentrates.

EXAMPLE GRASP RUN - Input data

Site factors

Grass area (hectares)	30
Annual rainfall (mm)	750
Main soil type	Clay loam
Grass species	Satisfactory
Proposed N use (kg per ha)	150 (and 250)
Normal grazing season	20 April to 25 October

Proposed stocking

18-month beef

Turnout weight (kg)	180
Daily gain expected (kg)	0.8
Proposed turnout date	20 April
Number turned out	100
Change in numbers	15 July
Number after change	80

Ewes

Body weight (kg)	70
Turnout date	22 May
Number turned out	150
No change in numbers	

Lambs

Turnout weight (kg)	10
Daily gain (kg)	0.2
Turnout date	22 May
Number turned out	225
Change in numbers	10 June
Number after change	200
Change in numbers	26 June
Number after change	150
Change in numbers	15 August
Number after change	100
Change in numbers	15 Sept
Number after change	50
No other changes	

EXAMPLE GRASP RUN - Output data

Potential
stocking rate

kg/ha	1,341.00	Average stocking rate
lu/ha	2.88	for grazing season

silage potential tonnes	grazing ha needed	area needed for grazing in each sixth of the season at potential stocking rate
98.88	11.96	
74.21	18.48	
12.62	27.24	
-10.75	32.94	
-21.79	36.36	
-12.27	33.16	

silage 1st five sixths-tonnes	153.16	surplus assumed to be silage and likely yields shown

This shows that silage can be made in the first half of the grazing season but that there is insufficient grazing later . Repeat calculation with N increased.

Nitrogen/ha
    250.00   ***   Increase nitrogen from 150 kg/ha

Potential
stocking rate
    kg/ha   1,810.35
    lu/ha   3.89

    silage   grazing
    potential   ha
    tonnes   needed
    156.44   8.66
    141.36   13.63   Output shows adequate
     68.58   20.18   grazing throughout
     27.62   24.40   grazing season and
     14.19   26.93   400 tonnes of silage
     28.51   24.56

Silage 1st five
sixths-tonnes   400.19

RESULTS in 1982

During the 1982 grazing season 333 areas of grassland were recorded in more detail than usual by members of the BEEFPLAN and FLOCKPLAN schemes (Spedding, 1983). This allowed overall stocking rates to be related to annual rainfall, soil type and grazing or conservation management. Variations in stocking over the season were also recorded.

There was a wide variation both in overall stocking and the way stocking varied through the season. Figure 1 shows the pattern of stocking through the grazing season on units achieving average and top third stocking rates.

Top third stocking rates were 450, 760 and 450 kg liveweight per hectare higher than average in May, June and July respectively, but the difference was less in August, September and October (360, 225 and 80 kg)

Differences in stocking patterns due to annual rainfall and soil type were less than would be expected from the ADAS/GRI GM 20 trials (Morrison et al,1980)

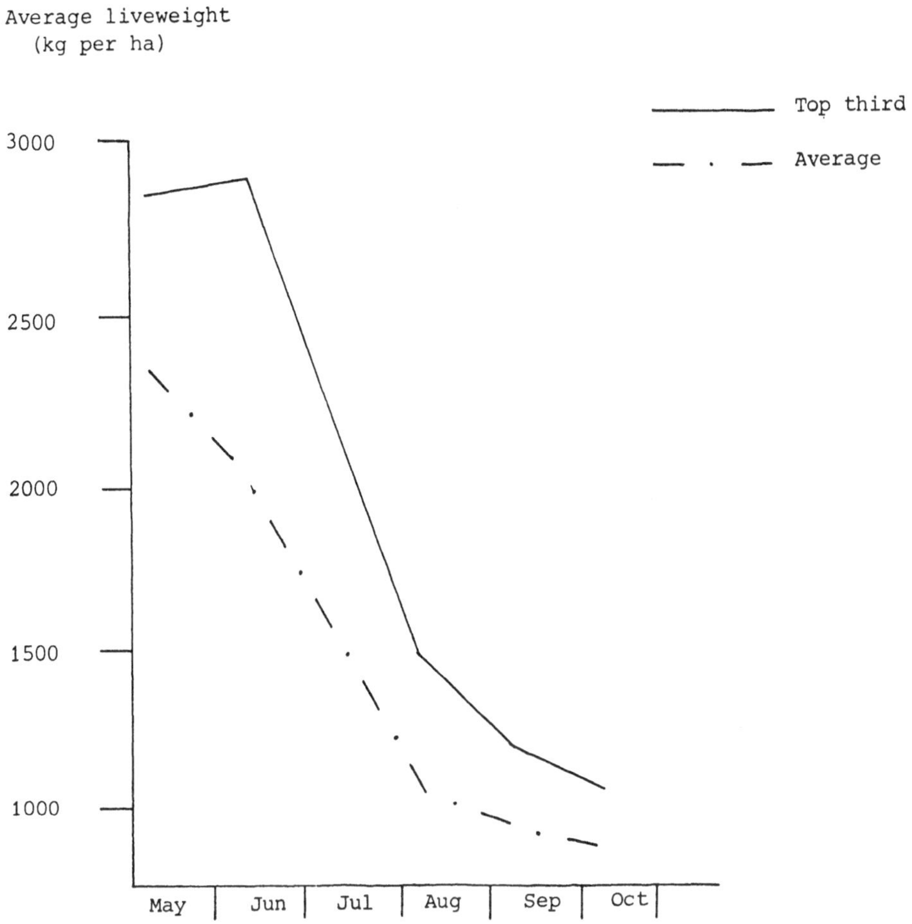

Average liveweight
(kg per ha)

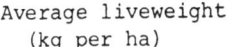

Fig. 1   Average and top third stocking rates at 200 kg N per ha

Figure 2 shows the pattern of stocking on units with different soil types.

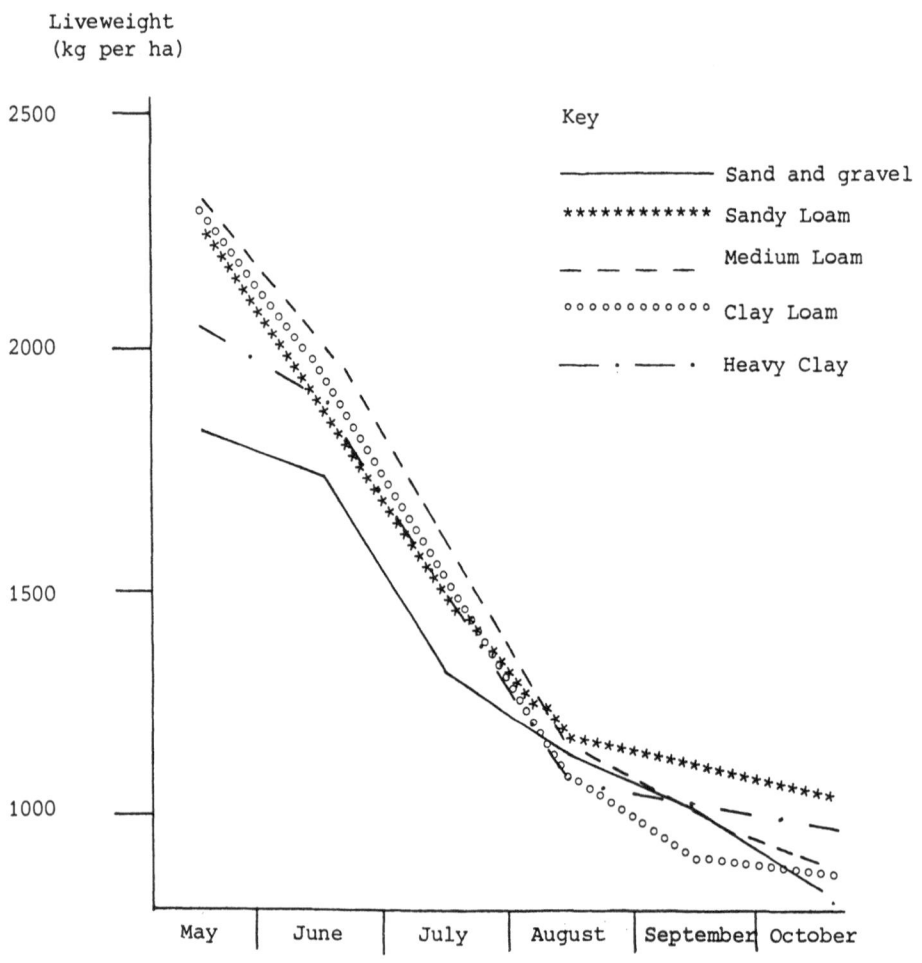

Fig 2 Stocking rates and soil type

Only sand and gravel soils have a markedly different pattern of stocking, though heavy clay soils tended to be more lightly stocked than others during May and June.

Figure 3 shows no effect of annual rainfall in level of stocking, except perhaps on units in the wettest areas which tended to have lower stocking rates early in the season.

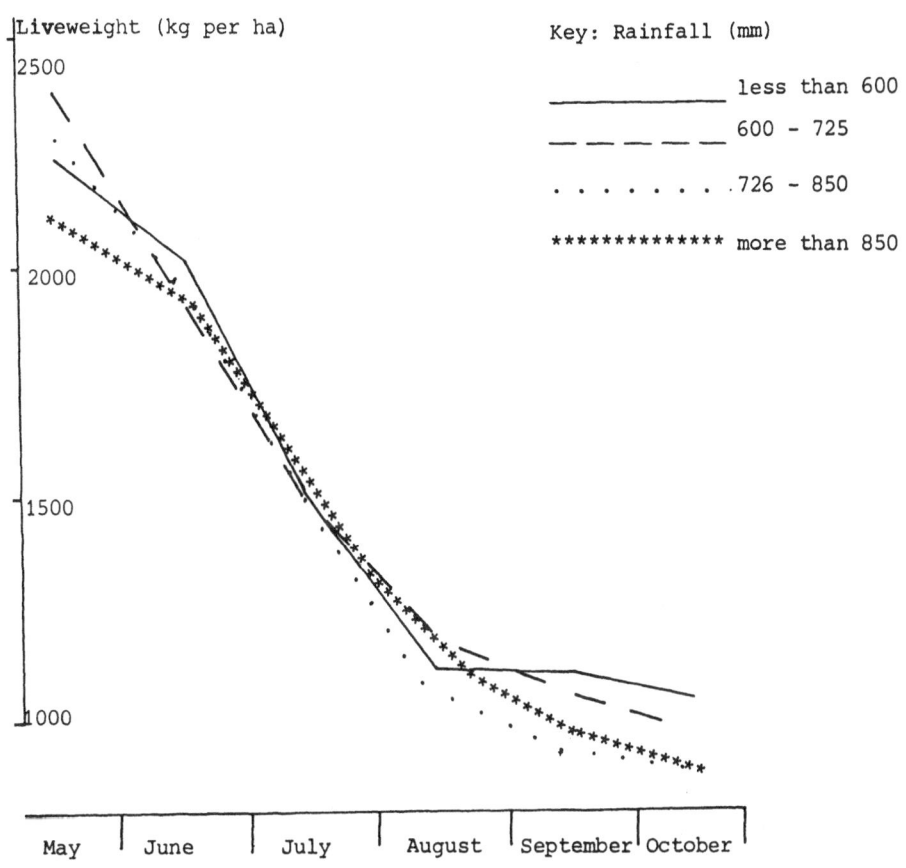

Fig. 3 Stocking rates and rainfall

58

Figure 4 compares stocking rates on 45 areas of grassland where more than 90 per cent of the utilisation was as silage with 56 grazed areas where there was no conservation. Silage made was converted to its equivalent as liveweight stocked per ha.

Liveweight (kg per ha)

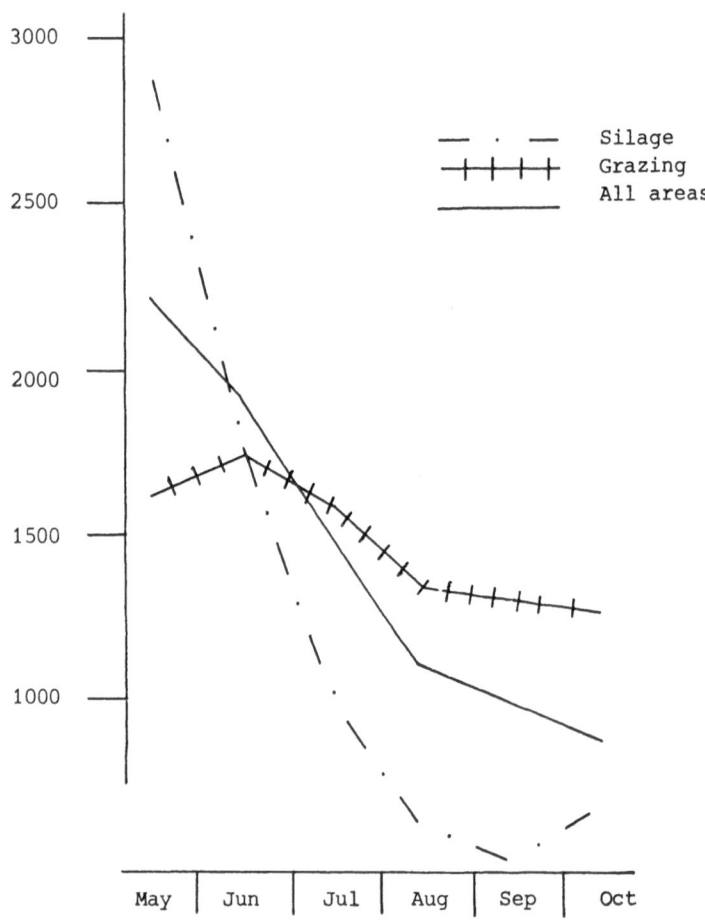

Fig. 4   Stocking rates on conservation-only and grazing-only areas

Patterns of stocking were very different from the all-areas pattern. Silage areas had a level of production in the first two months of the season equivalent to a higher stocking rate than grazed areas, but thereafter production from silage areas was lower.

Grazed areas showed much more level stocking through the season than silage areas or areas on which grazing and conservation were integrated.

CONCLUSIONS FROM 1982 RESULTS

Care needs to be taken in drawing conclusions from one year's records especially since 1982 was a good grass year in most areas of Britain, which may have masked differences in stocking due to annual rainfall and soil type. However, it seems likely that inputs used in GRASP will need modification to be less influenced by notional site factors and more influenced by records of previous levels of stocking and by whether the swards concerned are to be grazed or cut for silage.

REFERENCES

Morrison, J., Jackson, M..V., and Sparrow, P.E. (1980). The response of perennial ryegrass to fertiliser nitrogen in relation to climate and soil. Report of the joint ADAS/GRI Grassland Manuring Trial —GM 20. GRI, Hurley.

Spedding, A.W. (1983). Data sheet 83/1. Meat and Livestock Commission, PO Box 44, Milton Keynes, UK

THE GRASSLAND REQUIREMENTS OF DIFFERENT BREEDS
IN BEEF PRODUCTION SYSTEMS

J.R. Southgate and A.W. Spedding
Meat and Livestock Commission,(MLC), PO Box 44, Queensway House,
Bletchley, MK2 2EF, UK

INTRODUCTION

The influence of breed on beef production in the UK is quite marked and a large number of sire breeds, with very different production characteristics, are used. The choice of beef breed varies both in suckler and in dairy herds. Farm recording schemes operated by MLC have shown consistent sire breed effects across different production systems (Allen and Kilkenny, 1980). In general the larger sire breeds produce faster growing progeny which are slaughtered at higher ages and heavier weights.

There is general agreement with the UK farm results in trials overseas (Smith,Laster,Cundiff and Gregory, 1976 and Bech Andersen,Liboriussen, Kousgaard and Buchter, 1977). In the UK, a basic understanding of the characteristics of the different sire breeds has often led to management practices being tailored to particular breeds, thus modifying the breed effects in farm results. For instance, it is normal to feed European continental breed crosses a higher quality ration in the knowledge that they will not become over-fat at unduly light weights. In the absence of reliable information on feed intake and carcase composition, MLC set up the Beef Breed Evaluation Programme in the early 1970s. Suckled calves were finished in both winter and summer feeding systems at MLC's Ingliston unit, and dairy bred cattle were reared on 16 and 24 month systems at the Sutton Bonington unit. Cattle were fed a complete diet to facilitate feed recording. In the first phase of these trials animals were slaughtered at a fixed depth of subcutaneous fat (see Southgate, Cook and Kempster, 1982a; Kempster, Cook and Southgate, 1982a,for dairy bred beef systems; and Southgate, Cook and Kempster, 1982b; Kempster, Cook and Southgate, 1982b,for suckled calf finishing systems)

Implications of sire and dam breeds in suckler finishing systems are discussed in relation to the total feed requirements of suckler systems by Southgate (1982). Differences in feed efficiency in suckler finishing systems were small. Although progeny sired by the large Charolais breed required 33 per cent more feed to produce a given amount of saleable meat than those sired by the smaller Angus, when the total feed requirement of the breeding cows and the finishing system were considered the Charolais crosses required 10 per cent less feed than the Angus crosses per kg of carcass produced.

This paper seeks to use the results of the MLC Beef Breed Evaluation Programme for dairy bred calves to determine the grassland requirements of different breeds in relation to the grassland planning method proposed by Spedding (1983). Consideration is given to Friesian, Hereford and Charolais cross Friesian cattle which are numerically important, yet markedly different in production characteristics. Friesian and Holstein bulls accounted for 62 per cent of the AI demand in the UK in 1981/82, most of the male progeny being available for beef production. Hereford and Charolais bulls accounted for 18 and 7 per cent of demand respectively and both male and female progeny contribute directly to UK beef production. The use of any other breed was insignificant in comparison to these three (Milk Marketing Board, 1982)

Breed effects

Results from the MLC Beef Breed Evaluation Programme single slaughter phase (Southgate et al.1982a) for these breeds are given in Tables 1 and 2.

Hereford x Friesian steers were about the same weight as Friesians at three months and had similar daily gains through to slaughter. However, they had lower feed intakes and were consequently more efficient. They were ready for slaughter about six weeks earlier than Friesians. Charolais x Friesian steers were heavier at three months and had higher daily gains to slaughter. Although their feed intake was also higher they were more efficient than Friesians. The Charolais crosses took two weeks longer than the Friesians to reach slaughter condition. The marked difference in age between the cattle in the finishing periods of the two systems did not affect relative breed performance.

These results have been used to deduce generally applicable performance and dry matter requirements for the three breeds in grass/cereal systems (Table 3).

The similarity in the relative breed results at daily gains ranging from 500 to 1000 g suggests that the data can be used with confidence in planning most grass/cereal systems, though still with some uncertainty about the possible effect of daily gain on rate of fattening; this subject is currently being investigated by MLC. For this paper finishing systems

TABLE 1
- Performance of Friesian, Hereford x - and Charolais x Friesian steers in the MLC Beef Breed Evaluation Programme 16-month system 1973-78

Breed	3 to 6 months			6 to 10 months			10 months to slaughter*			
	Start weight (kg)	Daily dry matter intake (kg)	Daily gain (g)	Start weight (kg)	Daily dry matter intake (kg)	Daily gain (g)	Start weight (kg)	Daily dry matter intake (kg)	Daily gain (g)	Number of days
Hereford x Friesian	89	3.8	873	187	6.5	936	293	8.0	741	143
Friesian	85	4.0	890	184	7.0	982	295	8.8	753	190
Charolais x Friesian	99	4.4	995	212	7.4	1038	329	9.6	850	213

* corrected to 6.7% estimated sub. fat content

TABLE 2
- Performance of Friesian, Hereford x - and Charolais x Friesian steers in the MLC Beef Breed Evaluation Programme 24-month system 1973-78

Breed	3 to 6 months			6 to 11 months			11 to 20 months (store period)			20 months to slaughter*			
	Start weight (kg)	Daily dry matter intake (kg)	Daily gain (g)	Start weight (kg)	Daily dry matter intake (kg)	Daily gain (g)	Start weight (kg)	Daily dry matter intake (kg)	Daily gain (g)	Start weight (kg)	Daily dry matter intake (kg)	Daily gain (g)	Number of days
Hereford x Friesian	86	3.3	768	158	6.6	939	290	8.4	500	447	12.1	996	50
Friesian	91	3.9	822	168	7.2	946	301	9.3	486	457	11.8	868	90
Charolais x Friesian	105	3.8	876	188	7.3	1045	334	9.6	569	517	12.2	1056	95

* corrected to 7.2% estimated sub. fat content

TABLE 3
- Relative performance of Hereford x - and Charolais x Friesian steers to Friesians in grass beef systems derived from MLC Beef Breed Evaluation Programme 16- and 24-month system results

(Friesian = 100)

	Start weight	3 to 12 months		12 to 18 months (store period only)		Finishing		
		dry matter intake	daily gain	dry matter intake	daily gain	dry matter intake	daily gain	period (days)
Hereford x Friesian	100	91	97	90	101	97	100	- 44
Charolais x Friesian	116	104	109	104	117	106	112	+ 14

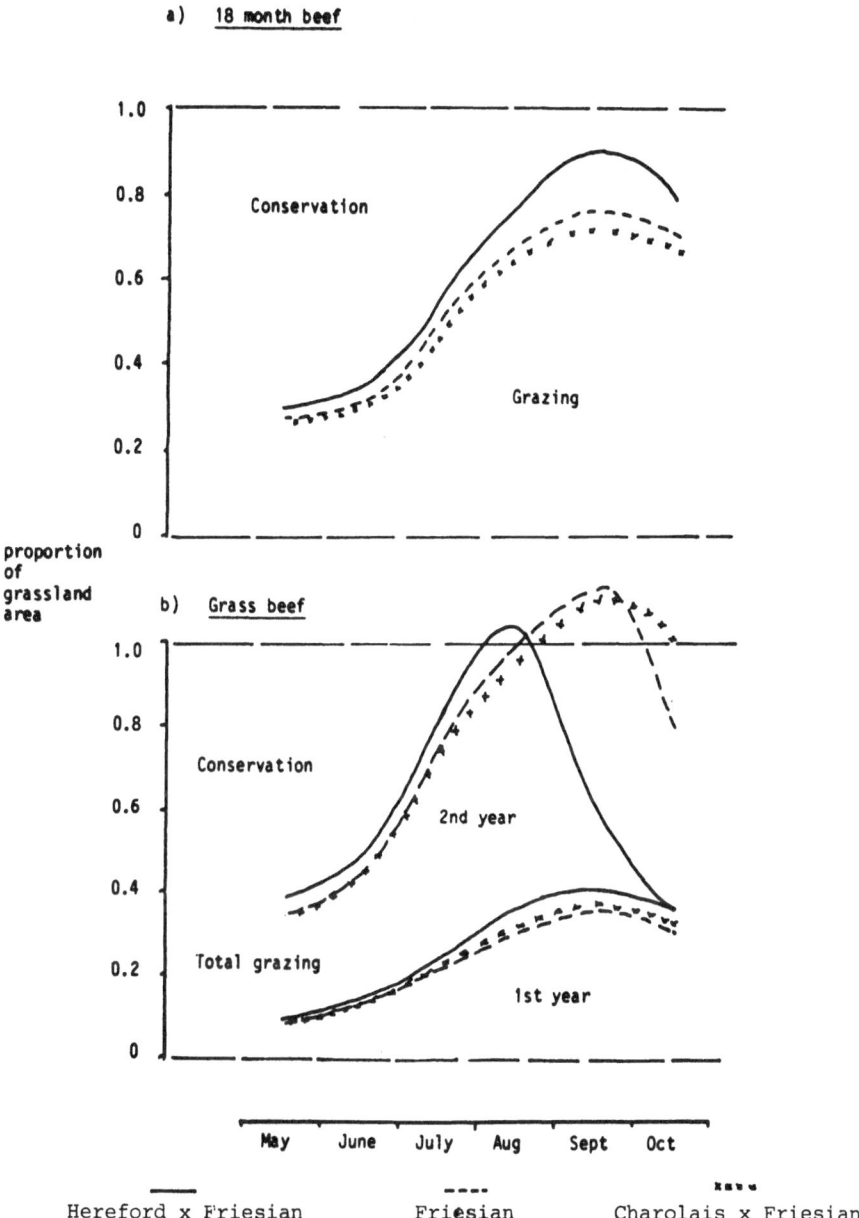

Fig. 1   Estimated grazing and conservation requirements for three
breeds in two grassland systems through the grazing season

with daily gains around 1000 g per day for Friesians have been chosen.

Grassland requirements have been calculated for two important systems, 18-month grass/cereal beef with winter finishing in yards and two-year grass-finished beef. Allen and Kilkenny (1980) have suggested performance targets for Friesian steers in these systems (Table 4) and feed requirements have been estimated to achieve these targets using the dry matter intakes in Tables 1 and 2.

TABLE 4 Target daily gains for Friesian steers (kg)

	18 month beef	grass beef
Rearing to 3 months	0.8	0.7
3 months to turnout	0.7	0.7
1st grazing season	0.85	0.7
2nd winter	0.85	0.5
2nd grazing season	-	1.0
Overall	0.8	0.7

Allen and Kilkenny, 1980

These estimates are given in Tables 5 and 6. Performance targets and feed requirements have been calculated for Hereford cross Friesians and Charolais cross Friesians, using the relative results in Table 3. It has been assumed that calves are purchased in September for the 18-month system.

Grassland planning

The planning method proposed by Spedding (1983) is based on calculating the grazing requirements of an animal of a known weight and performance monthly through the grazing season.The conservation requirements can also be calculated by an iterative process. An absolute value is then given to stocking rate by relating these requirements to potential grassland output in terms of rainfall, soil type, nitrogen application and grass species. This method has been used with the breed results in Tables 5 and 6 and with the grassland conditions described in Table 7, to estimate grassland requirements of the three breeds in the two systems.

The number of animals, and their grazing requirements matched to conservation needs,which could be accommodated on 50 hectares of the described grassland are given in Table 8 for both systems. The balance between grazing and conservation is shown diagramatically in Figure 1.

TABLE 5   Estimated feed requirement and performance per head for beef breeds in an 18-month grass/cereal beef system from 3 months using Beef Breed Evaluation Programme results and published target performance.

First winter	Friesian	Hereford x' Friesian	Charolais x Friesian
Start weight (kg)	100	100	166
days to turnout	128	128	128
daily gain (g)	700	679	763
turnout weight (kg)	190	187	214
total concentrate (kg)	320	291	333
total silage (kg)	947	862	985
Grazing			
days to yarding	183	183	183
daily gain (g)	850	824	926
yarding weight (kg)	345	338	383
total concentrate (kg)	80	73	83
grass dry matter (kg)	1208	1099	1256
Second winter			
days to slaughter	159	115	173
daily gain	850	840	952
slaughter weight (kg)	480	436	548
total concentrate (kg)	400	281	461
total silage (kg)	4253	2984	4905
Overall			
daily gain (g)	808	789	893
total concentrate (kg)	800	645	877
total grass dry matter (kg)	2509	2061	2729

NOTES: 1 concentrates and grass products fed in constant ratio within periods

2 concentrates assumed 860g/kg dry matter

3 silage assumed 250 g/kg dry matter

TABLE 6   Estimated feed requirement and performance per head for beef
breeds in a grass finishing system from 3 months using Beef
Breed Evaluation Programme results and published target

First winter	Friesian	Hereford x Friesian	Charolais x Friesian
Start weight (kg)	100	100	116
days to turnout	67	67	67
daily gain (g)	700	679	763
turnout weight (kg)	147	145	167
total concentrates (kg)	168	153	175
total silage (kg)	461	420	479
First grazing season			
days to yarding	167	167	167
daily gain (g)	700	679	763
yarding weight (kg)	264	259	295
total concentrates (kg)	100	92	104
grass dry matter (kg)	1124	1023	1169
Second winter (store period)			
days to turnout	182	182	182
daily gain (g)	500	505	585
turnout weight (kg)	355	351	401
total concentrates (kg)	182	164	189
total silage (kg)	5121	4609	5326
Second grazing season			
days to slaughter	174	130	188
daily gain (g)	1000	1000	1120
slaughter weight (kg)	529	481	612
total concentrate (kg)	0	0	0
grass dry matter (kg)	2044	1481	2341
Overall			
daily gain (g)	727	698	821
total concentrates (kg)	450	409	468
total grass dry matter (kg)	4563	3761	4961

NOTES: 1   concentrates and grass products fed in constant ratio within periods

2   concentrates assumed 860g/kg dry matter

3   silage assumed 250g/kg dry matter

TABLE 7 Grassland conditions used in example

Annual rainfall 600-725 mm		Basic stock-carrying capacity 1360 kg liveweight/ha
		Adjustment factors
Soil type	medium loam	1.01
Nitrogen	200 kg/ha	1.18
Grass species	broad leaved	1.00
Estimated stock-carrying capacity of 50 ha		81,040 kg liveweight

DISCUSSION

The results of this study suggest that different grassland management should be adopted for the two systems. In the 24-month system, grazing demand is higher at turnout and rises more sharply, so that a lower proportion of grassland is available for conservation. The model suggests that it is more difficult to balance grazing and conservation needs in the 24-month system and in this example a period of grass deficit is indicated for all breeds. This could be an important management factor. For the 18-month system the apparent constant conservation allocation provides a buffer against a poor season, but this is not available in the 24-month system. A shortage of grazing may require expensive concentrate feeding, whereas a shortfall in conservation can be accommodated by modifying the winter feeding strategy. Thus it is common practice to reduce total fodder required in finishing systems by increasing daily gain with additional concentrates. This reduces the length of the finishing period and in itself limits both forage and total concentrate use.

The results suggest that breed type should also influence strategy. The higher grassland conservation requirements for later maturing breeds in the 18-month system, caused by the longer winter finishing period suggest a lower grazing allocation. Although the difference is only four per cent of the grassland area at the beginning of the season it becomes fifteen per cent in the late summer. The later maturing breeds also require conservation in late season, while two cuts will be adequate for the Hereford crosses. On the other hand, because the Hereford crosses require to graze most of the grassland area in the late season, the provision of grazing for these cattle is likely to be more critical.

TABLE 8   Estimated annual stocking and monthly grazing requirement on 50 hectares grassland for three breeds in two beef systems

	18 month beef			Grass beef		
	Friesian	Hereford x Friesian	Charolais x Friesian	Friesian	Hereford x Friesian	Charolais x Friesian
No of animals sold	146	177	132	88	103	86
Stocking rate (hd/ha)	2.9	3.5	2.6	1.8	2.1	1.7
Grazing requirement (ha)						
May	13	15	13	17	19	17
June	15	17	14	22	24	22
July	26	29	25	37	42	37
Aug	34	39	33	49	54	48
Sept	39	45	36	56	31	55
Oct	35	40	34	40	18	49

In the 24-month system the requirements of the breeds are reversed. The early slaughter of the Hereford relieves the pressure on grass production in the late summer and autumn. However, this may not always be an advantage. A significant proportion of the conservation for the early maturing breed is required from late season grass. Apart from the difficulty in maintaining grass quality in this period, any delay in slaughtering the early maturing animals will jeopardise the conservation allocation.

Both system and breed have significant effects on grassland utilisation. This paper has of course studied only a few of the possible management systems: thus feed requirements and the balance of grazing and conservation can be changed by the alteration of the time at which calves are purchased; while the effects of concentrate feeding, growth rate and fat deposition are further essential components. These are being investigated in the final stages of MLC Beef Breed Evaluation Programme, and it is hoped that this model can be developed for wider application.

REFERENCES

Allen, D.M. and Kilkenny, J.B. 1980. Planned beef production. Granada Publishing : London

Bech Andersen, B., Liboriussen, T., Kousgaard, K. and Buchter, L. 1977. Crossbreeding experiment with beef and dual-purpose sire breeds on Danish dairy cows. III. Daily gain, feed conversion and carcass quality of intensively fed young bulls. Livest. Prod. Sci. **4** 19-29

Kempster, A.J., Cook, G.L. and Southgate, J.R. 1982a. A comparison of the progeny of British Friesian dams and different sire breeds in 16 and 24 month beef production systems. 2. Carcase characteristics and rate and efficiency of meat gain. Anim. Prod. **34** 167-178

Kempster, A.J., Cook, G.L. and Southgate, J.R. 1982b. A comparison of different breeds and crosses from the suckler herd. 2. Carcase characteristics. Anim. Prod. **35** 99-111

Milk Marketing Board. 1982. Report of the Breeding and Production Organisation, No. 32. MMB, Thames Ditton, UK

Smith, G.M., Laster, D.B., Cundiff, L.V. and Gregory, K.E. 1976. Characterisation of biological types of cattle. II. Postweaning growth and feed efficiency of steers. J. Anim. Sci. **43** 37-47

Southgate, J.R., Cook, G.L. and Kempster, A.J. 1982a. A comparison of the progeny of British Friesian dams and different sire breeds in 16 and 24-month beef production systems. 1. Liveweight gain and efficiency of food utilisation. Anim. Prod. **34** 155-166

Southgate, J.R., Cook, G.L. and Kempster, A.J. 1982b. A comparison of different breeds and crosses from the suckler herd. 1. Liveweight growth and efficiency of food utilisation.. Anim. Prod. **35** 87-98

Southgate, J.R. 1982. The current practice of commercial crossbreeding in the UK with particular reference to the effects of breed choice. In: Beef production from different dairy beef crosses. Current topics in veterinary medicine and animal science. Edited by G.J. More O'Farrell, published by Martinus Nijhoff for the Commission of the European Communities, **21** 333-358

Spedding, A.W. 1983. GRASP - a grassland planning programme for the HP41C programmable calculator. This publication.

EFFECT OF GRAZING METHOD, NITROGEN LEVEL, SUPPLEMENTARY FEEDING AND STOCKING RATE ON THE PERFORMANCE OF YOUNG GRAZING BULLS*

J.M. Bienfait[1], M. Gielen [1], P. Limbourg[2] and C.van Eenaeme[1]

1. Faculté de Médicine Vétérinaire, 45 rue des Vétérinaires,
      1070, Brussels, Belgium
2. Faculté des Sciences Agronomiques, 59 avenue de la Faculté,
      5800 Gembloux, Belgium

* Research supported by the IRSIA (Institut pour l'Encouragement de la
      Recherche Scientifique dans l'Industrie et L'Agriculture)

ABSTRACT

In 1981 and 1982 an experiment on beef production on pasture with growing fattening young bulls was started on permanent pastures situated on the plateau of the Belgian Ardennes. Rotational grazing and set-stocking were compared in association with the following factors: stocking rate, energetic concentrate supplement level and N-fertilizer intensity.

As a result of the high stocking rate (3209 kgLW/ha on average) and the excellent individual performances, weight gains from 1300 to over 1700 kg per hectare were observed. Performances were similar for the two grazing systems but rotational grazing required about 40% less fertilizer N per ha. Increasing the stocking rate by 32% (7.1 to 9.35 bulls/ha) resulted in higher weight gains per hectare with a concentrate supplement (+ 32%) than with an increase in N-manuring (+ 18%). Indeed in the former system weight gain per animal was maintained while it dropped by 11% in the latter. In the course of the grazing season it was more difficult to obtain good growth performances in mid-summer and in October shortly before the animals were removed from the pastures.

INTRODUCTION

Due to the climatic and pedological conditions in the south-eastern part of Belgium (Ardennes) permanent pastures play a dominant part in the economy of this region. Consequently farmers are concerned to improve management performances and to obtain both high individual performances per animal and per hectare.

From 1968, experiments were conducted with dairy cows to study the effects of an increase in stocking rate by raising the level of supplement feeding or of nitrogenous fertilizer or of both, in order to increase the production per hectare without impairing the individual milk production per cow (Limbourg et al.,1980; Bienfait et al., 1981; Gielen et al., 1982)

In 1980, in parallel with these dairy cow experiments, similar trials were started on beef production on pasture with growing fattening young bulls. Indeed, few experimental results are available on beef production on pasture in regions similar to the Belgian Ardennes and the few data relate to steers, while it is well known that performances obtained with post-pubertal entire male cattle (bulls) are distinctly superior to those obtained with castrated animals due to the presence of lower concentrations of endogenous sex steroids following castration (Reyneke, 1976; Roche et al.,1981; Gregory and Ford, 1983). Furthermore most of these publications studied one factor at a time,e.g. the effect of stocking rate,nitrogen fertilizer level or concentrate feed. Other experiments compared different management techniques such as limited grazing, rotational grazing or set-stocking.

In our work, these different factors and techniques were compared in a single experimental design repeated over several years. The present report deals with the results of the first two years (1981 and 1982)

EXPERIMENTAL

Pastures

The experimental site is located at the Ardennes plateau, about 500m above sea level. Local mean rainfall is high and regular (over 1000 mm/year). The pastures are permanent pastures, over sown in 1979 with a mixture of 20 kg/ha perennial ryegrass, 7 kg/ha timothy and 4 kg/ha white clover.

Animals

On 25 May, 36 young bulls with weights around 315 kg in 1981 and 48 weighing about 260 kg in 1982, were grouped into 6 homogenous lots of 6 to 8 animals (Table 1). Each year the bulls,most of them of the Belgian Blue breed, were turned out early in May in order to be as much as possible in similar condition when constituting the experimental lots. All animals were treated routinely with an anthelmintic when turned out to pasture and during the grazing season.

Grazing management

The experimental design was set up to compare 3 set or continuous stocking and 3 rotational grazing groups. Different stocking rates were used in both systems (Table 1). Stocking rate was increased either by providing a concentrate supplement (lots 2 and 5) or by additional N-fertilizer (lots 3 and 6).

The concentrate, a 1:1 mixture of cereals and dried sugar beet pulp, was given daily to each group of animals. As the animal requirement increased and the available grass decreased, the supply of concentrate was

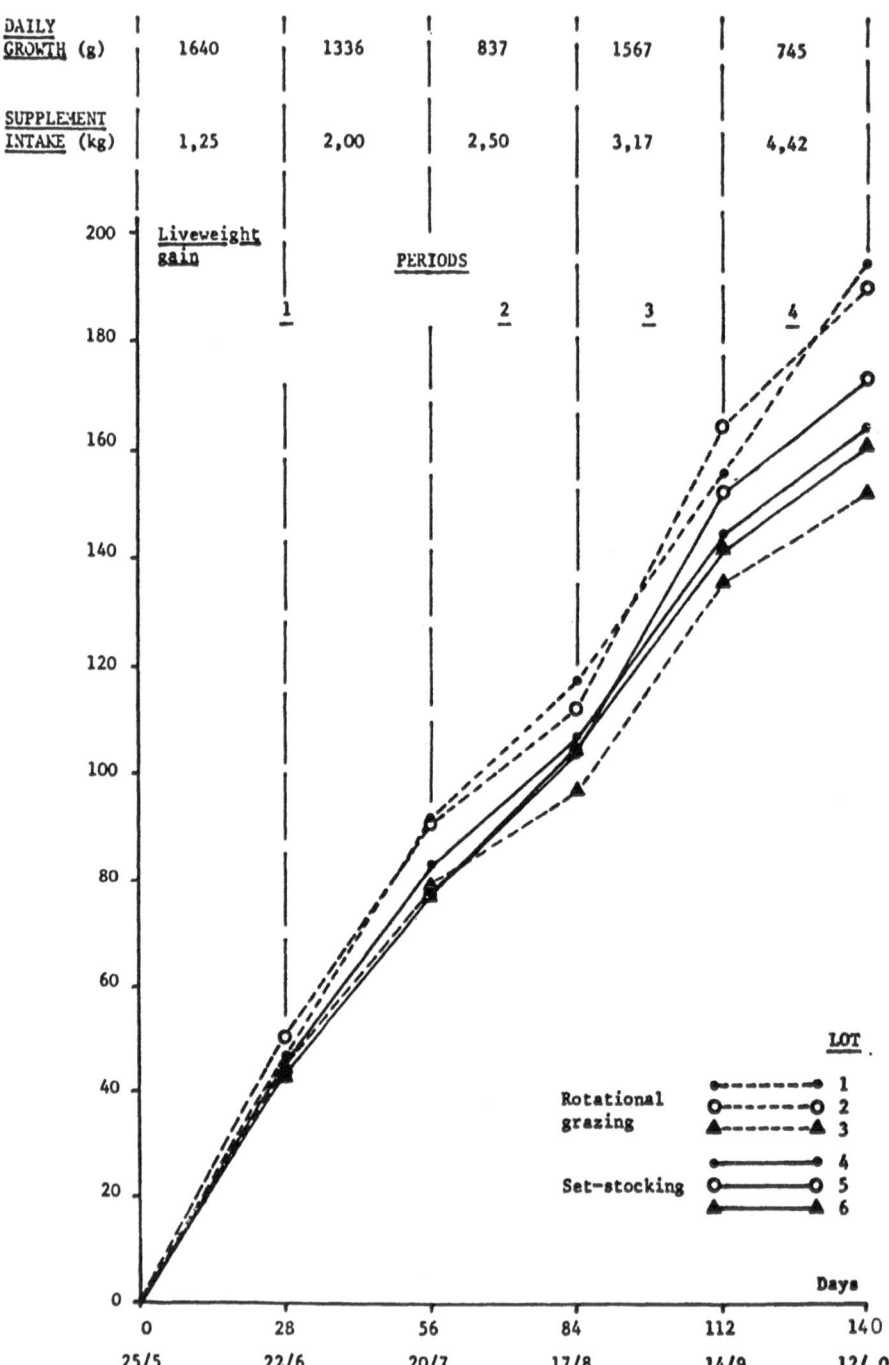

| DAILY GROWTH (g) | 1640 | 1336 | 837 | 1567 | 745 |
| SUPPLEMENT INTAKE (kg) | 1,25 | 2,00 | 2,50 | 3,17 | 4,42 |

Fig. 1   Evolution of liveweight gain (mean 1981 + 1982)
          daily growth and supplement intake for the different
          periods

TABLE 1   The experimental treatments

	Lot	Area of pasture allotted	Stocking rate bulls/ha 1981	1982	Feed supplement	N Fertilizer level
Rotational	1	5 x 0.15 ha	6	8	Low	Low
grazing	2	5 x 0.20 ha	8	10.67	High	Low
	3	5 x 0.20 ha	8	10.67	Low	Medium
Set Stocking	4	0.75 ha	6	8	Low	Low
	5	1.00 ha	8	10.67	High	Low
	6	1.00 ha	8	10.67	Low	Medium

increased.   The amount of concentrate was fixed monthly after a double weighing of the animals and determination of the daily growth obtained in the preceding period. A minimum daily growth of 1 kg during the entire experimental season was imposed.

Similarly, N-fertilizer was given in relation to the individual requirements of the different paddocks, in order to secure both an adequate supply of grass and to avoid excess grass growth which could be detrimental to its quality. Consequently, the N-fertilizer level was determined by the available amount of grass, which could differ from system to system.

RESULTS

Starting on 25 May, the lengths of the two pasture seasons were respectively 147 days in 1981 and 154 days in 1982. The evolution of total growth (mean of the two years) for the different treatments is shown in Fig. 1.   These results indicate that the experimental season (limited to the common period of 140 days) can be divided into 4 parts: (1) an initial period, when growth rates were high and similar for the different treatments: however the high growth rate obtained during the first month could partly be ascribed to compensatory growth after the winter season and also to a weight increase of the digestive tract (2) a second period, about mid-summer when growth rates decreased (3) a third period when growth rates rose again for all lots, while differences between treatments become more marked and (4) a final period, corresponding to the end of the season which is less important for this type of animal production particularly since supplement feed intake is relatively high at this time.

The actual stocking rates achieved per ha were in fair agreement with the experimental plan and were identical for the set stocking and rotational grazing systems at 8.6 young bulls per hectare. Table 2 shows these stocking rates (bulls/ha and kg LW/ha) together with the N-fertilizer

TABLE 2   Effect of different treatments on animal performance
(mean 1981-1982)

| Lots No. | Rotational grazing | | | | Set-stocking | | | |
	1	2	3	Mean	4	5	6	Mean
Actual stocking rate (Bulls/ha)	7.1	9.3	9.4	8.6	7.1	9.4	9.3	8.6
Initial liveweight (kg)	283.1	287.1	291.2	287.1	286.1	290.2	292.6	289.6
Final liveweight (kg)	479.5	477.1	452.2	469.6	461.0	470.1	462.5	464.6
Mean total weight/ha (kg)	2662	3503	3463	3209	2618	3549	3460	3209
N fertilizer (kg N/ha)	50	50	140	80	100	100	215	138
Feed supplement intake (kg/ha)	2394	5376	3565	3778	2394	5441	3533	3789
Feed supplement (kg/bull/day)	2.275	3.827	2.502	2.868	2.275	3.827	2.502	2.868
Grazing days/ha	1067	1405	1423	1298	1067	1423	1405	1298
Liveweight gain/ha (kg)	1365	1736	1509	1537	1237	1698	1559	1498
Daily liveweight gain (kg)	1.309	1.266	1.072	1.216	1.163	1.195	1.131	1.163

and concentrate levels applied and the animal performances recorded (number of grazing days/ha, liveweight gain in kg/ha and daily growth per animal). Over the two years 1981 and 1982 very satisfactory performances were observed: daily growth near 1200 g and weight gain per ha over 1500 kg, for a concentrate supplement intake under 3 kg per animal per day and a N-fertilizer level of 100 kg N per ha.

At identical stocking rates, comparison of rotational grazing and set stocking reveals a slight but non-significant advantage in weight gain per hectare, in favour of the rotational grazing system (+2.6%). This superiority of the rotational system is entirely due to the results obtained in 1981 (+ 10.8%) and in 1982 the set stocking gave slightly better results (+4.1%). While average concentrate intake was the same in both systems (2.87 kg/day), the application of N-fertilizer was substantially lower with the rotational grazing system, allowing savings of about 40% of N in both years.

To measure the effect of an increase in stocking rate achieved either by concentrate or N-fertilizer, the results were grouped across the different management systems (Table 3). For an identical rise in stocking

TABLE 3   Effect of grazing intensities on animal performance

	Low stocking rate	High stocking rate		General mean
		+ feed supplement	+N supplement	
Lots	1 + 4	2 + 5	3 + 6	
Actual stocking rate (bulls/ha)	7.1(100)	9.35(132)	9.35(132)	8.6
Mean total weight/ha (kg)	2640	3526	3461	3209
N fertilizer (kg N/ha)	75	75	177	109
Feed supplement intake (kg/ha)	2394	5408	3549	3784
Feed supplement (kg/bull/day)	2.275	3.827	2.502	2.868
Grazing days/ha	1067(100)	1414(132)	1414(132)	1298
Liveweight gain/ha (kg)	1301(100)	1717(132)	1534(118)	1517
Daily liveweight (kg)	1.236(100)	1.231(100)	1.102(89)	1.190

rate (32%) and consequently in grazing days, differences in weight gain per hectare were observed between the two systems. With the concentrate supplement system (lots 2 and 5) individual animal performances were maintained at the level of lots 1 and 4 (1230 g growth/day) resulting in a proportional (32%) rise in weight gain per hectare. On the contrary with the N-fertilizer a deterioration of individual performances (more than 10%) could not be avoided, so weight gain per hectare was increased by only 18% (lots 3 and 6). In 1982 it was even necessary for these lots to increase the concentrate supplementation in order to avoid a fall in daily growth below 1 kg/day, the limiting minimum value chosen in the experimental plan.

Increasing stocking rate from 7.1 to 9.35 bulls/ha by increasing concentrate supplement indicated that 416 kg extra weight gain per hectare was obtained with 3014 kg additional concentrate, i.e. 1 kg weight gain per 7.2 kg concentrate supplement. If a similar allowance is made for the additional concentrate used on the nitrogen treatment compared with the control the response to the nitrogen was 0.73 kg gain per kg N.

DISCUSSION

The performances obtained with young bulls on herbage in the Ardenne region during the years 1981 and 1982 compare favourably in liveweight production per ha (1500 kg/ha) with results in neighbouring countries (Table 4). These high yields are due to several factors: firstly, they are obtained with intact male animals whose performances are superior to those of steers or female animals of the same weight and age. Animals in perfect health (free of respiratory or parasite problems) should achieve good weight gains when they are offered a high quality young grass supplemented with a minimum amount of energetic concentrate feed. Chemical analysis confirms that digestibility (OMD : 79.9; D-value : 71.5;and energetic value (980 VEM,1617 Kcal or 6.77 MJ net energy per kg) and protein content (190 g DCP/kg DM) of the grass was very high. Addition of dried sugar beet pulp and cereals could consequently result in an improvement of the diet only by introducing additional carbohydrates (e.g. starch and pectins) because the protein requirements are already covered by the grass. Considering the high stocking rate (3200 kg/ha on average) high beef production per hectare can be obtained by maintaining the individual performance at a high level over the entire experimental season. However, in both years, at two distinct periods in the season a fall in performance was observed: first,in mid-summer, in a similar manner as observed by Andries et al,(1973) without however explaining this diminution entirely by availability or quality of the grass; second, at the end of the season when climatic conditions are adverse for the animals, grazing time decreases and feed efficiency drops. Consequently, this period is less valuable particularly since it is not possible to finish these bulls on herbage (Beranger, 1975)

In this experiment maintaining individual performances was easier with a concentrate supplement than with an increase in N-fertilizer to obtain higher grass yields. Positive responses to concentrate supplement for increasing stocking rate have been observed by Tayler and Wilkinson (1972)

TABLE 4   Comparative performances of beef cattle on pasture in Western Europe

Reference	Experimental site	Stocking rate cattle per ha	Initial liveweight kg	N applied kg/ha	Feed supplement level kg/day	Liveweight gain kg/ grazing ha	Grazing season No. of days
Alder et al 1967	UK	3.31-9.36	353-388	0-672	-	360-946	162-190
Andries et al 1973	BELGIUM	4.70-7.30	513-523	100-300	-	518-750	114-129
Boucqué et al 1978	BELGIUM	4.30-9.20	480	60 after each rotation	0-9.26	507-1302	118-133
Elliott et al 1978	UK	Mean 9 years 3.97	230-300	125-244	0.5-1.5 from late August	497-674	203
Elliott & Dale 1980	UK	4.11-3.52	280-350	140-190	-	509-908	April-November
Escuder et al 1971	UK	6.40-12.60	233-294	150-450	2;5 after 12 weeks	849-1260	168
Groot de & Keuning 1968	The Netherlands	?	294-317	204-611	-	721-1042	± 6 months
Holmes & Lang 1974	UK	Mean 11 years 3.70-4.80	330	51-263	-	569-683	144-184
Horton & Holmes 1974	UK	5.00-12.30	±200	50-504	-	630-1362	168
Lestang & Mourier 1981	France	Mean 8 years 5.2	301	196	-	687	206
	France	Mean 3 years 3.50-3.60	410	133-145	-	425-465	192
Marsh & Murdoch 1974	UK	5.00-7.50	139-263	400-800	-	1130-1264	168
Meadowcroft & Altman 1982	UK	4.13-12.35	196	63-375	-	588-900	154-182
Müller & Berenger 1978	France	6.50-3.40 spring-autumn	380	160	3	917	124
Umoh & Holmes 1974	UK	5.90-11.90	304 Average wt 255-333	50-329	-	547-1037	84 12 weeks
Yiakoumettis & Holmes 1972	UK	5.90-11.90		50-300	-	593-1005	140 20 weeks
Bienfait et al 1983	Belgium	7.10-9.40 8.6	283-293 288	50-215 109	2.4-5.4 3.8	1237-1736 1517	147-154 150

and Conway (1968). Vadiveloo and Holmes (1979) reported that concentrate supplementation was valuable when the quantity of grass available is low but the benefits of supplementation were low when grazing conditions were good, because the grass intake was then decreased. In our experiment the effectiveness of the supplement is explained rather by a better quality of the diet than by a lack of grass.

Increasing the N-fertilizer increased weight gain per hectare by about 18% but resulted in lower individual performances (11%) as observed also by Holmes and Lang (1974). However Umoh and Holmes (1974) and recently Meadowcroft and Altman (1982) report different results when studying grazing intensity and fertilizer level.

The two grazing systems (rotational and set-stocking) gave very similar performances per animal as was observed by Horton and Holmes (1974) and Vadiveloo and Holmes (1979). These two grazing techniques result in differences in grass growth physiology bringing about differences in N-supplies from one system to the other for the same quantity of grass available. Over the two years the rotational grazing system allowed N-fertilizer savings of 40% as was observed in our former experiments with dairy cows. This observation might be of importance when establishing a comparative balance of the two systems over several years.

REFERENCES

Alder, F.E. Cowlishaw, S.J., Newton, J.E. and Chambers, D.T. 1967
    The effect of level of nitrogen fertilizer on beef production from
    grazed perennial ryegrass/white clover pastures.
    J. Br. Grassld Soc. **22** 230-238.

Andries,A.P., Carlier, L.A., Boucqué,Ch.V.,Cottyn,B.G. and Buysse,F.X.
    1973. Production de viande bovine sur des prairies exploitées d'une
    manière intensive.
    Rev. Agric. **26** 1049-1061.

Béranger, C. 1975. La Complémentation au pâturage des bovins de
    boucherie. Fourrages, **62** 57-72

Bienfait, J.M.,Gielen,M. and Limbourg,P.1981. Exploitation des pâturages
    par la vache laitière dans les Ardennes Belges. Comptes rendus "Les.
    Entretiens de Bourgelat", Lyon, Oct. 1981, Edts Point Vétérinaire,
    tome 1 pp. 207-213

Boucqué,Ch.V.,Cottyn,B.G.,de Brabander,D.L.,Fiems,L.O.and Buysse,F.X.1978
    Effect of ad libitum energy supplementation to finishing steers on
    pasture. Proceedings of the 7th General Meeting of the EGF,Gent,
    Belgium, 5-9 June 1978 pp. 5.55 - 5.63

Conway, A.1968. Grazing management in relation to beef production. Effect
    of feeding supplements to beef cattle on pasture at two intensities of
    stocking. Ir. J. Agric.Res., 7 105-120.

Elliott, J.G.,Dale, R.J. and Barnes, F. 1978. The performance of beef
    animals on a permanent pasture. J. Br. Grassld Soc. **33** 41-48.

Elliott, J.G. and Dale,R.J. 1980. Further experiences of beef production on permanent pasture in 1976-1978. Grass and Forage Science, 35 319-321.

Escuder, J.C., Andrews, R.P. and Holmes, W. 1971. The effect of nitrogen, stocking rate and frequency of grazing by beef cattle on the output of pasture. J. Br. Grassld Soc. 26 79-84.

Gielen, M., Limbourg,P., Bienfait, J.M. and Van Eenaeme,C.1982. Continuous and rotational grazing management with dairy cows: comparison at two stocking rates. 9th General Meeting of the European Grassland Federation:Reading, 5-9 September, 1982.

Gregory, K.E. and Ford,J.J. 1983. Effects of late castration, zeranol and breed group on growth, feed efficiency and carcass characteristics of late maturing bovine males. J. Anim. Sci. 56 771-780.

Groot de Th. and Keuning, J.A. 1968. Intensive beef production from grassland. Two grazing experiments. World Review of Animal Production, 4 (18) 75-76.

Holmes, J.C. and Lang, R.W. 1974. The effect of nitrogen application to pasture on beef production. J. Br. Grassld Soc. 29 121-131

Horton, G.M.J. and Holmes, W. 1974. The effect of nitrogen, stocking rate and grazing method on the output of pasture grazed by beef cattle. J. Br. Grassld Soc. 29 93-99.

Le Stang, J.P. and Mourier, C. 1981. Utilisation des prairies permanentes normandes pour la production des boeufs de races laitières. Fourrages n° 86, 49-80.

Limbourg, P., Noirfalise, A., Bienfait, J.M. and Gielen, M. 1980. Nitrogen manure and concentrate feeding : two methods to increase the pasture stocking rate for grazing dairy cows. Ann. Med. Vet. 124 497-513.

Marsh, R. and Murdoch, J.C. 1974. Effect of high fertilizer nitrogen and stocking rates on liveweight gain per animal and per hectare. J. Br. Grassld Soc. 29 305-313.

Meadowcroft, S.C. and Altman, Jill F.B. 1982. Nitrogen and stocking rates for grazing beef cattle. Expl. Husb. 38 163-183.

Muller, A. and Beranger, C. 1978. Production de jeunes boeufs à partir d'herbe verte ou ensilée complémentée avec des pulpes séchées. Bull. Techn. CRZV, Theix, INRA, 31 5-9.

Reyneke, J. 1976. Comparative beef production from bulls, steers and heifers under intensive feeding conditions. S. Agr. J. Anim. Sci. 6 53-58.

Roche, J.F., Harte, F.J., Joseph, R.L. and Davis, W.D. 1981. The use of growth promoters in beef production. Proceedings of a Workshop held at Brussels,24-27,March 5-6th,1981,CEC.

Tayler, J.C. and Wilkinson,J.M. 1972.The influence of level of concentrate feeding on the voluntary intake of grass and on liveweight gain by cattle. Anim. Prod. 14 85-96.

Umoh, J.E. and Holmes, W. 1974. A further investigation of the effect of nitrogen and stocking rate on the productivity of pasture for beef cattle. J. Br. Grassld Soc. 29 203-206.

Vadiveloo, J. and Holmes, W. 1979. Supplementary feeding of grazing beef cattle. Grass and Forage Science 34 173-179.

Yiakoumettis, I.M. and Holmes, W. 1972. The effect of nitrogen and stocking rate on the output of pasture grazed by beef cattle. J. Br. Grassld Soc. 27 183-191.

ALL GRASS BEEF

E.H. Glover

Edinburgh School of Agriculture, West Mains Road, Edinburgh,Scotland

ABSTRACT

Although many British beef cattle on 18-month systems consume 500-1000 kg of concentrates, consideration of their energy requirements and of the energy value of conserved forages indicates that beef production on grazing and forage alone is technically feasible.

A trial was conducted to compare the lifetime performance of a total of 72 Sussex x Friesian steers and heifers, born in either autumn or spring, fed grass silage ad libitum with no supplement or with 2-3 kg barley/day during the winter period and grazed during summer.

The supplement resulted in small but significant increases in daily gain of 0.055 kg/day and of 6.9 kg in carcase weight. Costings indicate that the all grass and forage treatment would yield the greater margin per head, under a wide range of cost/price structures.

This trial is seen as a physical model of one of many possible "all grass" beef systems. A mechanistic model is required to identify the most appropriate system for a specific farm.

INTRODUCTION

The 18-month system of beef production is characterised by a daily liveweight gain from weaning to first turnout to pasture of 0.7 kg/day and 0.8 kg/day thereafter. Concentrate feeding during winter may reach a maximum of 5 kg/head/day, leading to a usage of about 1 tonne of concentrate during the lifetime of the animal.

Calculation of the energy requirements of cattle following the 18-month system suggests that the minimum Metabolisable Energy density required for the diet is of the order of 9-10 MJ per kg dry matter. Good quality grass silage and grazed grass have an energy density of this order, or better, suggesting that a substantial input of concentrates is unnecessary.

Figure 1 summarises a range of experiments reviewed by Wilkinson (1979) where grass silage was offered ad libitum with only limited concentrates. He noted gains of 0.71 to 1.14 kg/day. None of these trials, nor those of McIlmoyle (1978) or of Broadbent (1977) considered the entire production cycle.

A trial conducted at Wye College (University of London) specifically examined the lifetime performance of Sussex x Friesian steers and heifers born in either autumn or spring and fed ad libitum grass silage and zero or 2-3 kg of barley during the housed period, (Glover, 1982)

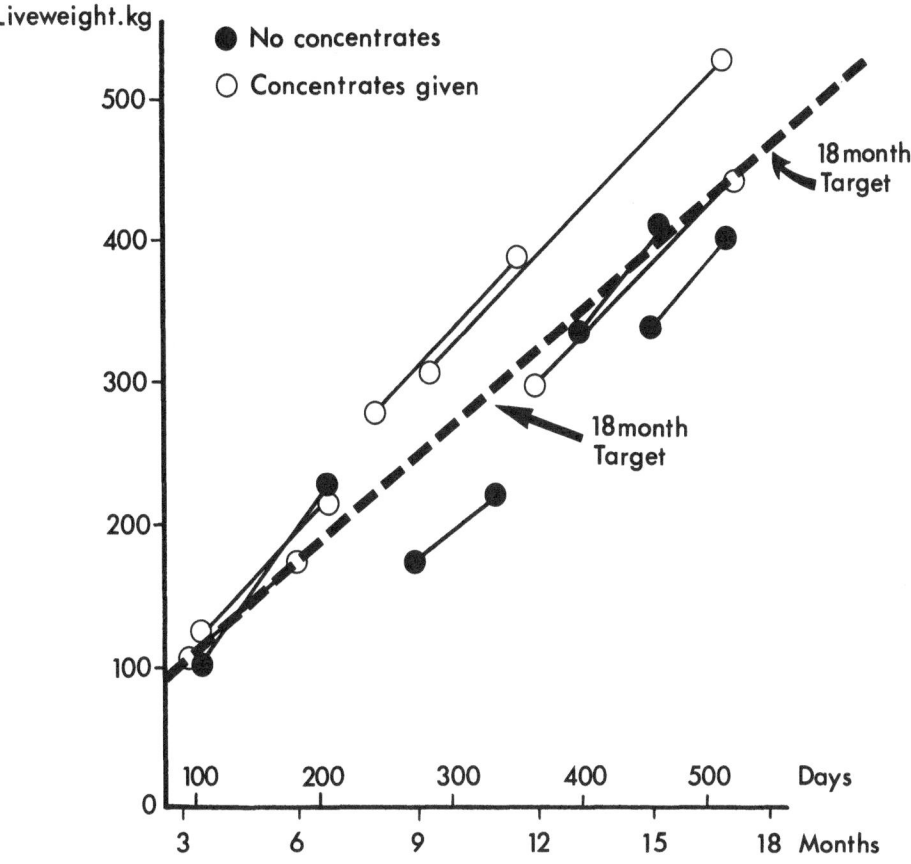

Fig. 1 Performance of cattle on grass silage and low concentrate levels

PRINCIPLES OF TRIAL WORK

In an investigation of this sort it is important to consider the nature of the general question asked. By definition an experiment answers a specific question. It is a qualitative assessment from which a conclusive answer should result. An experiment should say "YES" or "NO" to a hypothesis. If it says "PERHAPS" or "SOMETIMES" it is a trial, not an experiment.

The experiments summarised in Figure 1 lead us to believe than an adequate growth rate can be obtained without concentrate usage. We seek in this trial to discover the truth of this. If adequate performance is not achieved we shall not conclude that concentrates are always essential, we shall instead find some reasons, less politely called excuses, for failure. The trial is a physical model of a method of beef production.

To analyse trial results the requirement is to summarise the performance of cattle, and correct the results for the factors which we believe to be responsible for differences between individuals or sub-groups. Any remaining differences we may then ascribe to the imposed treatment. Multiple regression is appropriate here since this will also overcome statistical problems caused by unbalanced numbers of replicates in sub-groups.

The fundamental assumption in analysing trial work is that we understand the mechanisms at work and that we can identify the important factors. We must continually question this assumption and if we find cause to doubt the mechanism then we should conduct experiments to clarify the doubt. A trial is useful in testing our understanding and in pinpointing our ignorance.

METHODS

The trial began in autumn 1977 and the last cattle were slaughtered in spring 1981. Five separate batches of cattle were recorded during this period, three autumn born and two spring born. Each batch was composed of approximately equal numbers of Sussex x Friesian steers and heifers and these were in turn divided into two treatment groups to be referred to as grass and control. The intention was to have 16 cattle in each group subdivided into 4 sub-groups of 4, but the actual number of cattle in any sub-group varied from 3 to 5. In total 72 cattle were recorded. The imposed treatments were different management strategies. Control cattle were offered concentrates according to normal practice for an 18-month beef system, that is, a level of 2-3 kg of rolled barley during the winter period, and 0.5, rising to 1.5 kg during the six weeks at pasture before yarding. Grass cattle were offered minimal concentrates as calves and at first turnout, and none thereafter up to slaughter. Good quality grass silage from the same clamp was offered ad libitum to both groups of cattle from soon after weaning. The cattle grazed together on the same pastures.

Differences in ages of cattle and general circumstances resulted in differences in time of imposition of treatment and of general management tactics. The pattern of management of each group of cattle is shown in Figure 2. Hatched areas indicate periods when the control cattle were receiving concentrates. Shaded areas indicate when cattle were grazing. The sloping ends of the bars show the buildup of batches and the rate of removal by slaughter.

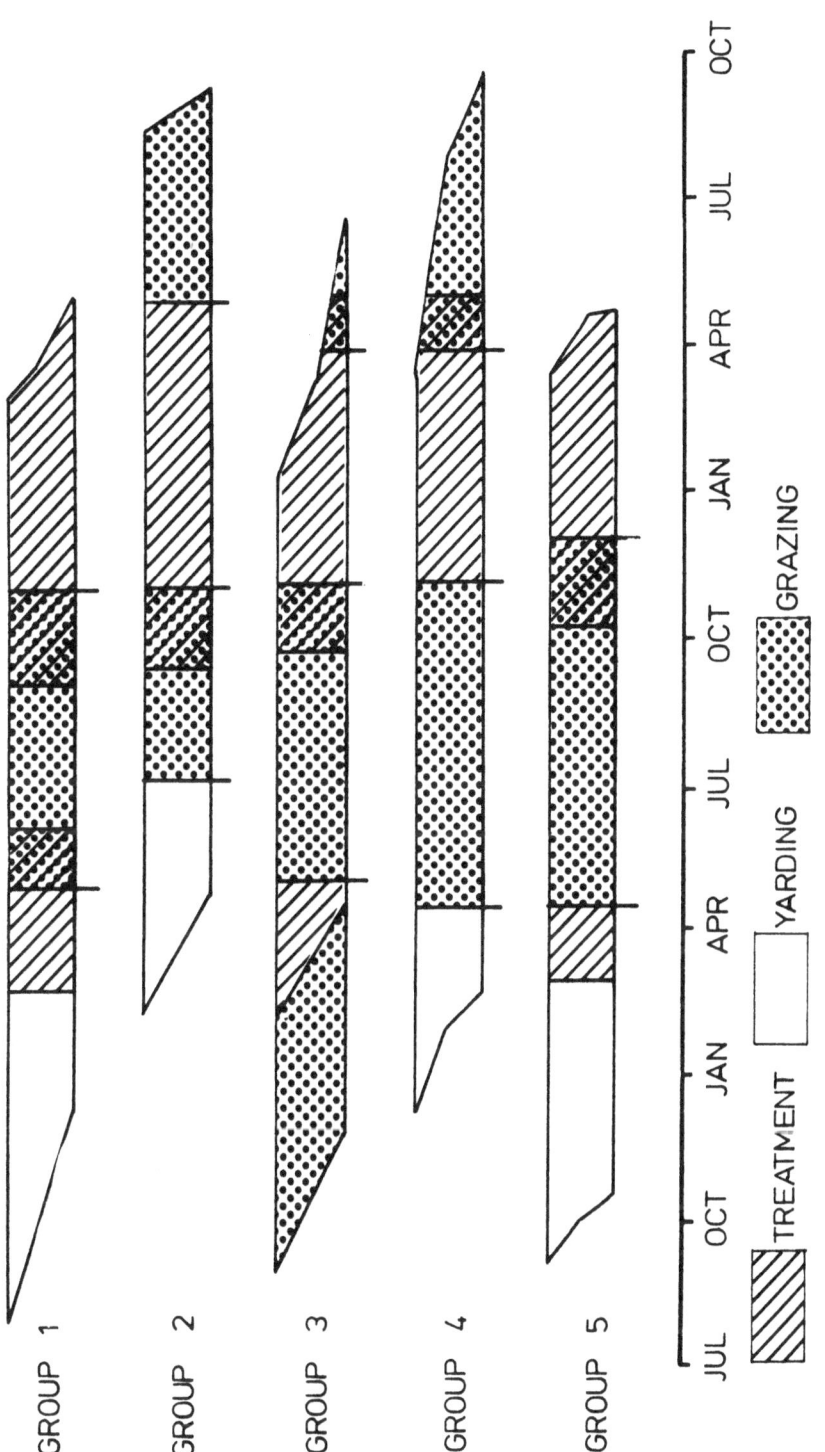

Fig. 2 Comparative management patterns

Groups 1,3 and 5 were autumn born and were divided into treatment groups for a period prior to first turnout. Group 1, control cattle, received concentrates for a period after turnout. Spring born cattle, that is Groups 2 and 4, received the same treatment until the end of their first summer. Cattle in Group 2 received some concentrates before yarding but the supply of grass to cattle in Group 4 was such that no concentrates were felt to be necessary. All spring born cattle were slaughtered from grass in the subsequent year, while all except two of the autumn born cattle were finished on winter diets.

Cattle were weighed weekly from approximately 8-10 weeks old onwards, and detailed records were kept of all management changes and levels of feeding. The target fat class at slaughter was equivalent to 4L on the EEC Beef Carcass Classification Scale. Target liveweights of 450 kg for steers and 420 kg for heifers were used to select cattle for slaughter, although cattle were occasionally slaughtered at other weights if handling indicated that they were unlikely to achieve the target fat class at the target weight. Cattle were weighed before dispatch to the abattoir where carcasses were weighed hot and assessed for fatness and conformation by MLC staff, using the MLC classification.

ANALYIS OF RESULTS

Liveweights

The mean daily liveweight gain for each animal was derived by linear regression of the recorded weights upon time. The mean values are presented in Table 1. The mean daily liveweight gain of all cattle was 0.78 kg/day which compares with the target of 0.8 kg/day. The differences between sexes and between treatments are shown in Table 2. Heifers gained 0.084 kg/day more slowly than steers while the control cattle grew 0.055 kg/day faster than those on the grass treatment. Although these effects are as expected, they are surprisingly small. The small treatment effect suggests that some compensation may have occurred between various points in the growth path of the cattle. Variation in management pattern and feed quality was found to result in some differences between groups, although liveweight gains of the 5 groups were not significantly different from each other and there were no significant differences between spring and autumn born cattle.

TABLE 1 Liveweight gains (kg/day) by regression

	PERIOD 1	PERIOD 2	PERIOD 3	PERIOD 4	LIFETIME
	1st weighing to 1st turnout	1st turnout to yarding	Yarding to Slaughter/ 2nd turnout	2nd turnout to slaughter	
Group 1	0.93	0.90	0.99	-	0.81
Group 2	1.00	0.89	0.87	1.18	0.78
Group 3	0.91	0.97	0.79	0.92	0.85
Group 4	0.80	0.82	0.83	0.75	0.75
Group 5	0.69	0.65	1.09	-	0.70
Steers	0.87	0.86	0.98	1.06	0.81
Heifers	0.86	0.83	0.87	0.96	0.75
'Grass'	0.85	0.86	0.85	0.99	0.75
'Controls'	0.88	0.83	1.00	1.04	0.81

The lifetime of each animal may be divided into four periods, where period 1 is from first weighing to first turnout, period 2 is from first turnout to yarding, period 3 is from yarding to either slaughter or second turnout and period 4 is from second turnout to slaughter. Period 4 is applicable mainly to the spring born cattle. The propositions to be tested here are that steers will grow faster than heifers and that the possible compensation noted earlier will result in some periods when the cattle without barley will grow faster than those with barley.

TABLE 2 Factors affecting lifetime LWG (kg/day)

Sex	-0.084 ± 0.016	***	(ie.heifers slower growing)
Treatment	0.055 ± 0.016	***	(ie.controls faster growing)
Group	see text	***	

Table 3 shows the magnitude of the effects in each of the four periods. Calves are small in period 1, weighing on average 147 kg at the end of the period, and it is unlikely that differences in metabolism due to sex would be substantial. The only significant difference due to treatment occurred in period 3, the second housed period, when control cattle were receiving 2-3 kg of barley per head per day. There is no evidence of compensation in either of the two grazing periods. Separate analysis of spring and autumn born cattle resulted in similar conclusions.

TABLE 3   Factors affecting short term LWG (kg/day)

Effect	PERIOD 1 1st weighing 1st turnout	PERIOD 2 1st turnout to yarding	PERIOD 3 Yarding to Slaughter/ 2nd turnout	PERIOD 4 2nd turnout to slaughter
Sex	ns	−0.079 ±0.026 **	−0.081 ±0.033 *	−0.200 ±0.072 *
Treatment	ns	ns	0.153 ±0.032 ***	ns

Slaughter weights and ages

The slaughter results are shown in Table 4. The overall mean slaughter weight for the steers was 445 kg, which compares with the target of 450 kg, and for the heifers the actual weight was 414 kg which again compares with the target of 420 kg. No detailed analysis of the variation in fatness and conformation scores has been made, but 50% of all cattle were in the target fat class, and only 4% were more than one classification away from the target.

The liveweights at slaughter showed no treatment effects (Table 5). Thus if any treatment effects do exist they will be manifested by treatment differences in carcass weight.

Small differences in killing out percentage may be expected due to differences in conformation and due to the rate of gain. Conformation and age at slaughter were therefore included in the regression model. Table 6 shows the significant effects. Sex, group, conformation and age, all act as significant correcting factors in the expected direction. The conformation effect was 8.3 kg for each unit change on the 5-point scale of the Meat and Livestock Commission. There then remains a difference in the corrected carcass weight of 6.9 due to treatment.

TABLE 4 Mean weights and ages at slaughter

	Liveweight (kg)	Carcass weight (kg)	Age (days)	Carcass gain (kg/d)	Killing out percentage
Group 1	427	234.6	529	0.396	54.9
	±8.2	±5.6	±8.2		
Group 2	429	227.0	536	0.377	52.9
	±7.7	±15.2	±6.6		
Group 3	432	226.0	509	0.395	52.3
	±5.4	±3.3	±11.4		
Group 4	425	222.8	544	0.364	52.4
	±9.0	±4.1	±21.5		
Group 5	427	221.5	560	0.351	51.9
	±8.1	±4.9	±4.5		
Steers	445	235.7	533	0.395	53.0
	±4.9	±3.2	±7.6		
Heifers	414	218.5	536	0.361	52.8
	±3.1	±2.0	±6.9		
Grass	424	222.9	545	0.363	52.6
	±4.6	±2.4	±6.5		
Controls	433	230.6	525	0.392	53.3
	±4.9	±3.3	±7.6		

The distribution of fat classifications for the two treatment groups suggests that the control cattle were fatter. These are shown in Figure 3. The fatness classification is on the old Meat and Livestock Commission scale. Class 1 spans classes 1 and 2 on the EEC classification. It is quite apparent that the cattle in the control group are distributed more toward the fat end of the scale.

TABLE 5 Factors affecting liveweight at slaughter

Sex	−34.9 ± 5.6	***	kg
Group	−	***	
Conformation	8.3 ± 3.4	*	kg/unit score

TABLE 6   Factors affecting carcase weight

Sex	−21.0 ± 3.1	***	kg
Treatment	6.9 ± 3.1	*	kg
Group	−	***	
Conformation	8.3 ± 1.9	***	kg/unit score
Age	0.104 ± 0.040	*	kg/day

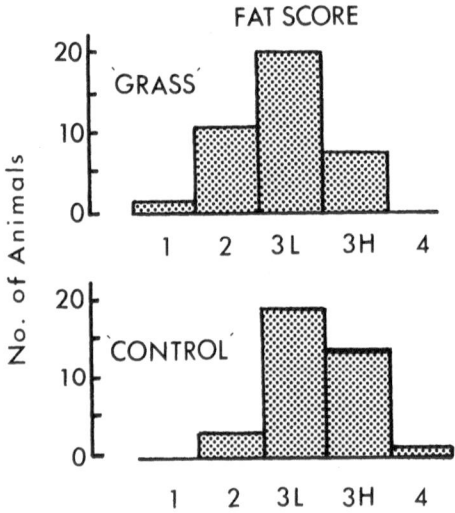

Fig. 3 Distribution of fat scores

Feed usage

A record was kept of the feed offered to each sub-group throughout, and these records were combined with the management record to produce a detailed outline of feed consumption by each animal excluding grazing. These in turn were aggregated to provide the mean estimates of feed usage by each sub-group shown in Table 7.

TABLE 7   Feed usage summary

	Misc concs kg as fed	Barley kg as fed	Silage + hay kg as fed	ME MJ	MJ/kg DM	Cost £/hd
Grass steers	79	16	3378	9577	10.21	32
Control steers	112	439	2767	13094	11.22	71
Grass heifers	66	8	3600	9815	10.19	31
Control heifers	99	416	2809	12799	11.19	67
All grass	72	12	3497	9705	10.20	28
All control	105	427	2789	12933	11.20	69
DIFFERENCES						
Steers	33	423	−611	3517	−	39
Heifers	33	408	−791	2984	−	36

The different management treatments led to the control cattle receiving approximately 450 kg more concentrates than the grass cattle, most of this difference being composed of barley. This extra concentrate feeding appeared to reduce silage intake by approximately 600 kg freshweight for steers and approximately 800 kg freshweight for the heifers. Overall, the steers on the control treatment received approximately 3.5 GJ more ME than the grass steers and for the heifers a similar difference of 3 GJ.

To explain growth of cattle a simple mechanism can be postulated. Firstly that growth is driven by body protein weight and protein supply. The energy in the diet is used firstly for maintenance, secondly for protein synthesis and thirdly the remainder is deposited as fat. Any deficiency of energy for protein synthesis is made up from fat reserves. It is assumed that protein supply is not limiting (Glover, 1983)

The difference in feed supplies to the two groups of cattle is equivalent to a feed with an energy density of about 15.5 MJ/kg DM and a Digestible Crude Protein Content of 80 g/kg DM. There is therefore likely to be a greater increase in growth of fat than of protein in the control cattle and therefore slaughter at a given weight results in control cattle being fatter than the grass treatment animals. This is of course what was observed.

Compensatory growth is also explained by this mechanism since the body fat is seen simply as a feed reservoir.

GRAZING PERFORMANCE

Cattle from different groups were grazed as one herd and different pastures were used at different times of the grazing season. Analysis of grazing performance is therefore restricted to summaries of combined performance of the groups grazing in each of the three years. The level of performance at grass was relatively low with a mean production of only 574 kg of liveweight gain per hectare per season. This is partly because cattle were slaughtered off grass in each season, leading to fairly light stocking in autumn. However it is clear that more intensive stocking would have produced better overall performance figures. Individual liveweight gains were generally good, averaging 0.68 kg per day over all cattle. (Table 8) Control cattle received approximately 90 kg per head of barley divided between the start and the end of the season. As was noted earlier, no differences in rate of liveweight gain were evident between the two treatment groups.

TABLE 8   Grazing performance

| | Year | | | |
	1978	1979	1980	Mean
Mean liveweight (kg)	200	255	303	254
Stocking rate/ha	4.3	6.6	4.1	4.9
Stocking weight (kg/ha)	868	1684	1251	1255
Supplementary conc. (kg/ha)	487	133	135	243
Nitrogen application (kg/ha)	100	200	80	125
Mean LWG (kg/d)	0.74	0.76	0.55	0.68
Production (kg/ha)	502	796	459	574

The grazing data are combined with estimates of the land area required to grow the supplementary barley and silage fed to give an estimate of the overall stocking rate of these control and grass groups of cattle (Table 9)

FINANCIAL PERFORMANCE

No attempt has been made to derive full gross margin budgets for the two treatments, but the differences in gross margin would be due to differences in feed costs and in carcass value. Therefore financial performance can be evaluated by estimating the margin of treatment feed costs over the carcass value. Table 10 shows that while the grass treatment animals produce carcasses of lower total value, this was offset by the reduced feed costs to a point where the grass animals showed an improvement in margin of £30 per head over the controls.

TABLE 9 Calculation of stocking rate, 'Control' animals

Grazing	0.2 ha for 150 days	= 30.0 hectare.days
Silage	2.8t @ 12.5 t/ha = 0.22 ha	
	0.22 ha for 60 days	= 13.2 hectare.days
Barley	0.5t @ 5.0t/ha = 0.10 ha	
	0.10 ha for 150 days	= 15.0 hectare.days
	Total	58.2 hectare.days

58.2 ha.d over 150 days   = 0.39 ha
Therefore overall stocking rate = 2.6/ha

'Grass' animals

Grazing	0.2 ha for 150 days	= 30.0 hectare.days
Silage	3.5t @ 12.5 t/ha = 0.28 ha	
	0.28 ha for 60 days	= 16.8 hectare.days
Barley	0.1t @ 5 t/ha = 0.02 ha	
	0.02 ha for 150 days	= 3.0 hectare.days
	Total	49.8 hectare.days

49.8 ha.d over 150 days   = 0.33 ha
Therefore overall stocking rate = 3.0/ha

Table 11 shows the difference in margins for each of the 5 groups. The difference in margin was much more variable for steers than for heifers but no clear explanation for this is apparent. In only one case were control cattle likely to be more profitable than the grass treatment sub-group. The grass treatment cattle were shown in Table 9 to require less land per head due mainly to their reduced requirement for barley. Offsetting this is their increased requirement for silage. It is therefore difficult to say which treatment will give the greater gross margin per hectare. Much depends on the opportunity cost of the grain on the farm.

TABLE 10   Partial budgets, overall costs returns and margins (£/head)

	Treatment feed cost	Carcass value	Margin (1) over treatment
Grass steers	32	342	310
Control steers	71	359	288
Grass heifers	31	307	276
Control heifers	67	315	248
(1) Margin over treatment = Carcass value - Treatment feed cost			

TABLE 11   Partial budgets,difference between margins over treatment(1)
(£ per head)

Group	1	2	3	4	5	All
Steers grass - control	-8	70	7	22	7	22
Heifers grass - control	10	30	34	30	27	28
(1) Margin over treatment = Carcass value - Treatment feed cost						

The partial budgets were based on the actual prices of the feeds and carcasses. A more general estimate of the financial benefits of the grass treatment is shown in Table 12. A saving of 450 kg of barley was offset by an extra consumption of 0.7 tonnes of silage, and by a reduction in carcass weight at slaughter of 7 kg. Taking the mean prices during the experimental period this equation estimates a financial improvement of £23.70 due to the grass treatment. This compares with the estimated mean improvement of £22 for steers and £28 for heifers.

TABLE 12   Theoretical saving under different price structures

	1978-1980 prices	1983 prices	extreme prices
Saving by Grass Treatment	= 0.45 x barley price	= 0.45 x £120/t	= 0.45 x £80/t
	-0.7 x silage price	-0.7 x £9/t	-0.7 x £20/t
	-7.0 x carcass price	-7.0 x 190p/kg	-7.0 x 250p/kg
Total saving	= £23.70	= £34.40	= £4.50

Taking 1983 prices as £120 per tonne for barley, £9 per tonne for silage and 180 pence per kg for carcasses, the financial improvement in present terms is £34.40. Examination of the variations in the saving achieved, when each of the prices rises by 10 per cent, shows that barley price is the dominant factor. It is apparent that the grass treatment will remain the most economic under a very wide range of conditions.

SUMMARY

To summarise, this exercise in physical modelling has demonstrated that omitting concentrates from the feeding regime of an 18-month beef system can lead to an overall financial improvement, and that this is likely to be valid under a wide range of feed costs.

By its nature and its role on farms, a beef system of any type is based on a series of marginal economic decisions. On a given farm, 3 influences that must be considered are:

(a) the quantity and quality of the basal roughage feed that is available
(b) the breed of cattle
(c) the price structure applicable to the year in which the decision has to be made

The best way that the beef system may be decided upon for a given farm in a given year is by using a conceptual model of a beef enterprise. Such a model must be capable of dealing with the biology of growth and development of cattle and of showing the economic implications of a given management decision. The model must also be capable of integrating the physical requirement, and financial performance of each of the groups of cattle present on the farm over a period of time, whether or not these different groups are following the same system. The development of such a model began at Wye College and has been continued at the Edinburgh School of Agriculture.

The financial support of the Meat and Livestock Commission during this work is gratefully acknowledged.

REFERENCES

Broadbent, P.J. 1977. A note on the effect of omitting the cereal
    supplement from a diet offered to weaned single suckled calves.
    Anim. Prod. **24** 275-278
Glover, E.H. 1982 . Some practical and theoretical aspects of intensive
    dairy bred beef systems. PhD thesis, University of London
Glover, E.H. 1983. Compensatory growth in beef cattle (Abstr.)
    Anim. Prod. **36** 516
McIlmoyle, W.A. 1978. Silage for beef production. In:An.Rept.Ag.Res.
    Inst.,NI.,No.51, 1977-1978,pp.20-24
Wilkinson, J.M. 1979. Realising the potential for animal production from
    grass. Presented at 13th Annual Conference, Reading University
    Agricultural Club, Reading, 7 February 1979.

PERFORMANCE OF BULLS AND STEERS UNDER SIMILAR FEEDING
AND MANAGEMENT CONDITIONS

F.J. Harte

An Foras Taluntais, Grange, Dunsany, Co Meath, Ireland

ABSTRACT

Work conducted in Ireland on the production of beef from bulls is reviewed. Bulls show greater rates of daily gain and greater carcass weights than steers slaughtered at the same age, provided they are well fed Their carcasses also give a greater yield of lean meat.

Care must be taken to minimise disturbances to their behaviour. Growth promoters may be used to increase the liveweight and carcass gain of steers but may affect their behaviour adversely.

INTRODUCTION

In the past it has been the practice to castrate male cattle for several reasons including (a) castrated cattle are more docile and more easily used for draught purposes (b) castrated cattle develop fatter carcasses than bulls and fat was a valuable source of energy for manual workers (c) castration prevented indiscriminate breeding. None of these reasons is now so important and beef production from bulls has been more widely practised.

Experiments on the production of beef from bulls conducted at An Foras Taluntais are summarised below.

Bull and steer performance

Bull beef production has been reviewed by Turton (1962,1969), Brannang (1966) and Harte (1966,1969). Experiments over 15 years (Collins, Harte, Conway, 1972; Collins and Harte, 1973,1974; Harte, Curran and Vial, 1965; Harte and Curran, 1967, 1972; and Harte 1966, 1969a, 1969b, 1970, 1973) show that bulls grow faster and yield heavier carcasses than similarly aged and managed steers. The difference in growth rate in favour of bulls over steers can vary but the base from which the comparisons are made is important and this often leads to confusion regarding the actual differences. Many reports refer only to liveweight but a preferable measure is carcass weight. However,it is often not economically feasible to measure carcass gain at pasture realistically because of the stage of growth and/or degree of finish. Indeed, estimating gain in very light carcasses may be of limited application.

Performance of bulls and steers at pasture

In most production systems cattle go to pasture for the first time between the ages of two (spring-born) and six months (autumn-born calves). Table 1 shows the liveweight performance of various groups of similarly managed bulls and steers for the first season at pasture. The performances for the second season at pasture are listed in Table 2.

TABLE 1   Initial liveweights and daily liveweight gains of bulls and steers during their first season at pasture

Breed	Animals/ treatment	Initial weight kg bulls	steers	Age at going to pasture days	Days at pasture	Av.daily gain kg steers	difference in favour of bulls %	Reference
1 Ch.	12	52	57	40	210	0.77	1.9	Harte (1973)
2 Sim.	12	53	54	40	210	0.69	3.4	Harte (1973)
3 Fr.	10	115	115	128	228	0.80	8.8	Harte et al (1965)
4 Fr.	10	105	106	115	236	0.82	6.7	Harte & Curran(1967)
5 Fr.	10	114	121	136	244	0.70	10.5	Harte(1969a)
6 Fr.	10	128	126	132	180	0.92	1.2	Harte et al (1965)
7 Fr.	10	119	118	136	228	0.73	4.8	Harte(1969a)
8 Fr.	10	148	147	174	218	0.81	7.9	Harte (1972)
9 Fr.	12	170	168	196	220	0.63	12.9	Roche (1973)

Ch = Charolais cross;   Sim = Simmental cross;   Fr = Friesian

As expected the difference in liveweight in favour of bulls was small when the first grazing season ended at approximately 8 months of age (first two comparisons, Table 1). The steers in these groups (Harte, 1973) were castrated at 3 months of age. The actual age at which bulls start to grow faster than steers is difficult to determine and is likely to be related to plane of nutrition. If, as suggested earlier (Harte, 1965), bulls do not show accelerated growth rate compared with steers until they reach a liveweight of 180 kg little difference between young bulls and steers can be expected at 8 months of age. With older animals going to pasture for the first season, the bulls mainly grew faster than steers, with a mean difference of 7.5 percentage units. (Comparisons 3-9, Table 1)

All the animals tested during their second grazing season (Table 2) were over one year of age. In eight comparisons bulls gained an average of 13.6% more than steers (Comparisons 1-8), and in one there was no difference in gain. In three comparisons (10-12), in which there was a 5.6% advantage in favour of steers, the animals were grazed at relatively high stocking rates over a long grazing season, and daily gains were all low over the last 50-60 days (Collins et al,1972; Collins and Harte, 1973,1974).

TABLE 2   Initial liveweights and daily liveweight gains of bulls and steers during their second season at pasture

	Animals/ treatment Breed		Initial weight kg bulls	steers	Age at going to pasture days	Days at pasture	Av.daily gain kg steers	Difference in favour of bulls %	Reference
1	Fr.	10	201	203	330	240	0.95	19.9	Harte(1969b)
2	Fr.	10	348	322	512	176	1.08	18.9	Harte(1969a)
3	Fr.	8	352	326	485	168	1.04	16.6	Roche et al,1981
4	Ch.	14	337	331	430	194	0.69	14.2	Collins & Harte (1973)
5	Ch.	8	367	339	485	168	1.09	13.1	Roche et al. (1981)
6	H.	10	212	207	330	240	0.97	10.6	Harte(1969b)
7	Fr.	12	431	394	566	105	0.68	8.3	Roche (1973)
8	Ch.	13	323	314	430	187	0.79	7.5	Collins & Harte (1974)
9	Sim.	13	295	291	430	187	0.90	0	Collins & Harte (1974)
10	Fr.	13	310	293	435	209	0.85	-1.1	Collins et al (1972)
11	H.	13	294	297	435	209	0.85	-3.8	Collins et al (1972)
12	Fr.	14	321	314	430	194	0.69	-11.8	Collins & Harte (1973)

H=Hereford cross;Sim=Simmental cross;Fr=Friesian cross;Ch=Charolais cross

It is difficult to ascertain the reasons for variations in performance at pasture. Price and Yeates (1969) are of the opinion that poor performance of bulls at pasture is not due to greater expenditure of energy in walking, excitation and aggressiveness and they express the view that plane of nutrition plays a major role. Certainly the results presented here (Tables 1 and 2) with some exceptions (Harte et al, 1965 and Collins and Harte, 1974) show that the difference in favour of bulls over steers tends to be greatest when daily liveweight gains are high.
Turton (1969) in his review and Beranger (1976) agree with this. The difference in favour of bulls was greatest where the animals were set-stocked and as far as possible, not restricted in feed intake. In the other experiments (Collins et al.,1973 and Collins and Harte 1973,1974) the animals were rotationally grazed and maintained at pre-determined stocking rates throughout the grazing season, irrespective of grass growth in that particular season.

Collins et al.(1977) noted that the general restlessness of bulls at pasture compared to steers was not reflected in reduced animal performance. Indeed,in Comparison 2 in Table 2 (Harte,1969a), although the Friesian bulls were 17 months of age on going to pasture for their second season and appeared much more restless than the similarly treated steers grazing with them, their mean daily liveweight gain for that grazing season (176 days) was 1.28 compared with 1.08 kg per head for the steers. Yet,it would have been difficult to convince producers that the steers were not doing better than the bulls because of their quieter disposition. It must be emphasised that these animals had ample supplies of high quality feed.If feed supply at pasture is restricted it is likely that bulls will further reduce this supply by trampling as a result of their general restlessness compared to steers. Weather conditions, paddock size and shelter are also likely to affect bull performance more than that of steers.

Carcass yield of bulls and steers

Comparison of bull and steer performance is easier to interpret where carcass yields are obtained since liveweight differences may not be a true reflection of performance; thus bulls may be restless before weighing and therefore may have less gut fill compared to steers. But this has not been verified and data in Table 3 show that in all trials bulls had superior carcass weights to similarly treated steers, the actual difference being greatest at the higher carcass weights.

TABLE 3 Carcass weights, actual and percentage differences in favour
of bulls, over similarly treated steers slaughtered at
the same age

Breed	Animals/ treatment	Carcass weight kg bulls	kg steers	Difference in favour of bulls actual kg	percent	Reference
Fr.	10	320	278	42	15.1	Harte (1969a)
Ch.	14	340	296	44	14.9	Collins & Harte (1973)
Fr.	8	353	310	43	13.9	Roche et al. (1981)
Ch.	8	377	335	42	12.5	Roche et al (1981)
Ch.	13	327	294	33	11.2	Collins & Harte (1974)
Fr.	10	220	201	19	9.4	Harte (1969a)
Fr.	10	234	215	19	8.8	Harte & Curran (1967)
Sim.	13	308	285	23	8.1	Collins & Harte (1974)
Fr.	10	216	208	8	3.8	Harte & Curran (1967)

Fr=Friesian:Sim=Simmental cross;Ch=Charolais cross

Lean meat production

Data in Table 4 emphasise the ability of bulls to produce lean meat
compared to steers. Lean meat is defined as total carcass weight less bone
and carcass fat, except fat remaining within the lean meat (Harte & Curran,
1967). The higher meat yields result from a combination of the higher
carcass weights and a higher percentage of lean meat in the carcass.Carcass
composition was determined as described by Harte (1969a). Steers had a
mean of 66.5 % lean meat in their carcasses and bulls averaged 72.4% (range
69.0 to 76.7%). The carcass composition for steers (range 64.1 to 68.7%)
agrees with our earlier work (Harte & Conniffe, 1967 and Harte, 1968) and
with that of Drennan et al (1981) for similar animals.

In some experiments the extra carcass weight and lean meat has been
obtained from bulls without extra feed (Harte, 1966) particularly where the
extra yield was small. But although lean meat is produced more efficiently
than fat it is unlikely that the differences reported in Table 4 were
obtained without extra feed. Therefore we must conclude that if bulls are
to show their extra potential over steers in carcass yield and lean meat

TABLE 4   Lean meat in carcasses and difference in favour of bulls over steers

Breed	Animals/ treatment	Lean meat in in carcass % bulls	steers	Weight of lean meat kg bulls	steers	Difference in favour of bulls kg	Reference
Ch.	14	76.7	68.7	261	203	58	Collins & Harte (1973)
Fr.	10	71.8	64.1	230	178	52	Harte (1969a)
Ch.	13	74.3	67.2	243	198	45	Collins & Harte (1974)
Sim.	13	74.2	67.6	228	193	35	Collins & Harte (1974)
Fr.	10	70.4	65.5	165	141	24	Harte & Curran (1967)
Fr.	10	69.0	66.2	152	133	19	Harte (1969a)
Fr.	10	71.1	66.2	154	138	16	Harte & Curran (1967)

Fr=Friesian;Sim=Simmental cross;Ch=Charolais cross

production they must be properly managed and given adequate feed on pasture as well as at other stages of the production cycle. In this there is considerable scope for using grass feeds. Thus in many of the experiments reported over 75% of the total animal production was obtained from grass and grass silage, as is also the case in the system of two-year old beef production recommended by our Institute (Harte, 1982).

Behaviour of bulls

There are few reliable research results on the behaviour of bulls, no doubt due to the difficulty of measuring differences. Research workers might start work on this subject expecting difficulties, influenced by the reports of the often lethal behaviour of breeding bulls which are normally kept under very restricted conditions. From our experience at Grange and with producers I have seen no evidence that bulls kept for beef production are a serious danger to man. However their behaviour, particularly at pasture, can cause considerable damage to their potential feed supply. Bulls aged 6 months or more that have been well fed previously can be restless for approximately one month after going to pasture. Their general behaviour is likely to be at its worst if the land is wet, if they have no shelter and are confused by electric fencing, if they are paddock grazed and if they are in large groups. If bulls had been in separate smaller groups before going to pasture this is also likely to increase general tension. In this respect it can often be difficult to re-introduce successfully a sick animal.

Experience at our Institute and of producers leads to the following recommendations on the management of bulls at pasture:

If possible animals should be mixed into their groups
before going to pasture.

Slatted floors and overhead electric wires in housing
can reduce problems.

Bulls should be set-stocked rather than paddock grazed.
This will reduce movement interference and probably
allow for increased shelter.

Bulls should always be provided with adequate supplies
of feed.

Numbers per group should be low, ideally probably 10,
and preferably not more than 30 animals.

Sick animals should be introduced into an area alongside
the main group and then re-introduced into the main
group when there is a management change,e.g.,if the
animals go to a fresh paddock.

The effects of growth promoters

No discussion of bull beef production at this time would be complete without some reference to growth promoters. Thus in an experiment using Charolais cross Friesians and pure Friesians, Roche, Harte, Joseph and Davis (1981) compared the performance of implanted steers with non-implanted steers and with bulls. The steers had been castrated at 5 months of age.

There were 48 animals (24 Charolais crosses and 24 Friesians) with six groups each of 8 animals. Two of the steer groups were implanted with resorcyclic acid lactone (Ralgro) and trenbolone acetate (Finaplix) at 15 months of age as they went to pasture for the second season. They were re-implanted with Finaplix and progesterone + oestradiol benzoate (Synovex-S) at approximately 20 months of age, at the start of the winter finishing period. At pasture all animals were run together in a single group and during the winter period they were housed on slatted floors in groups of 8 and fed silage plus concentrates. All animals were slaughtered at the same age (26 months).

The mean difference in final carcass weight between bulls and implanted steers was 18 kg (Table 5) while the difference between bulls and untreated steers was 43 kg. Growth promoters were therefore effective in raising the steer performance towards that of bulls, although in this experiment there was a suggestion (Roche et al, 1981) that the bulls' performance was somewhat lower than might normally be expected in the final finishing period.

TABLE 5 Mean initial liveweights, liveweight gains and final carcass weights of steers, implanted steers and bulls

	Steers	Implanted steers	Bulls
Initial weight (kg)	332	329	359
Liveweight gain (kg)	258	302	284
Carcass weight (kg)	322	347	365

These results suggest that at least part of the adverse effect of castration can be restored by the use of growth-promoters, McKenzie (1983) has suggested that bull performance can also be improved by growth promoters but this was not tested in this experiment. However the dangers of consumer resistance (if not ill-health) even to the present level use of growth promoters, and the possibility that the use of some products may be partially or totally prohibited in the future must be recognised.

While accepting that behavioural measurements are subjective, I believe that implantation of steers with growth promoters causes them, at least in certain circumstances, to behave more like bulls than steers. The later the period of implantation the greater this problem is likely to be.

Future research

Further research is needed to clarify the effect of age and weight of bulls going to pasture and in particular the influence of available feed supply on performance. A comparison of bulls and optimally implanted steers in behaviour, liveweight performance and ability to produce lean meat would be of interest. In this respect Drennan et al.(1981) reported an increase in lean meat in the carcass of 1.3 percentage units (mean of two experiments) after implanting with Ralgro plus Finaplix in the final 114 day finishing period. Our earlier study (Harte & Curran, 1972) using growth promoters which are no longer available, resulted in increased lean meat content of the carcasses. Martin & Stob (1978) also reported increased lean meat in the carcass as a result of implantation.

CONCLUSIONS

Bulls which spent either one or two seasons at pasture had heavier carcass weights and greater yields of lean meat than comparably fed steers slaughtered at the same age.

Differences in liveweight gain at pasture have nearly always been in favour of bulls unless restriction of feed had occurred at some stage when steer and bull performances at pasture were similar. Further work is needed on behaviour of bulls at pasture. The effects of group size, availability of feed, method of grazing, shelter and general disturbance need investigation. Research is also needed on the comparative performance and behaviour of bulls and implanted steers at pasture.

The use of the entire male is the natural and probably the most efficient way to produce beef. The use of steers, whether implanted or not, was devised by man; probably to his benefit in the past, but not necessarily so today.

REFERENCES

Beranger, C.1976. Beef production from pasture. In: Improving the nutritional efficiency of beef production. p 120-131. CEC Publ. No.EUR 5488e
Brannang,E. 1966. Lantbr.hogsk. Medd. A.52
Collins, D.P., Harte, F.H. and Conway, A. 1972. Anim.Prod. Res. Rept. p.30-31. An Foras Taluntais, Dublin
Collins, D.P. and Harte,F.J. 1973. Anim.Prod.Res. Rept. p.34-35 An Foras Taluntais, Dublin
Collins, D.P. and Harte, F.J. 1974. Anim. Prod. Res. Rept. p.20-21 An Foras Taluntais, Dublin
Collins, D.P., Drennan, M.J. and Flynn,A.V. 1977. Potential Irish grassland for beef production. Proceedings International Meeting on Anim. Prod. from temperate grassland. p.12-19 (Ed. B.Gilsenan). An Foras Taluntais, Dublin
Drennan, M.J., Roche, J.F. and L'Estrange, J.L. 1981. Ir. J. agric. Res. 20 113-123
Harte, F.J., Curran, S. and Vial, V.E. 1965. Ir. J. agric. Res. 4 189-204
Harte, F.J. 1966. Breed type, castration and plane of nutrition in calfhood as factors affecting efficiency in cattle production. PhD thesis, Trinity College, Dublin University
Harte, F.J. and Conniffe,D. 1967. Ir.J. agric. Res. 6 153-167
Harte, F.J. and Curran,S. 1967. Ir. J. agric. Res. 6 101-118
Harte, F.J. 1968. Ir. J. agric. Res. 7 149-159
Harte, F.J. 1969a. Ir. J. agric. Res. 8 293-305

Harte, F.J. 1969b. Six years of bull beef production research in Ireland. In: Meat production from entire male animals. p.153-171. (Ed.D.N. Rhodes), J & A Churchill, London

Harte, F.J. 1970. Some aspects of efficiency in beef production. Third Richards-Orpen Memorial Lecture, 28 pages. Ir.Grassld Anim.Prod.Assoc, Dublin

Harte, F.J. and Curran,S. 1972. Ir. J. agric. Res. 11 251-259

Harte, F.J. 1973. Anim.Prod.Res.Rept. p.20.An Foras Taluntais,Dublin

Harte, F.J. 1982. Anim.Prod.Res.Rept.(in press)An Foras Taluntais,Dublin

Martin,T.G. and Stob,M. 1978 . J. Dairy Sci. 61 104-105

McKenzie, J.R. 1983. N.Z. Vet.J. 31 104-105

Price, M.A. and Yeates, N.T.M. 1969. Growth rates and carcass characteristics in steers and partial castrates. In:Meat production from entire male animals. p.69-77 (Ed. D.N. Rhodes), J & A Churchill, London

Roche, J.F., Harte, F.J.,Joseph,R.L. and Davis, W.D. 1981. The use of growth promoters in beef production. p.27-44. Anabolic agents in beef and veal production. Proc. of EEC Workshop, Brussels, 5-6 March. Commission of the European Communities.

Roche, J.F. 1973. Personal communication

Turton, J.D. 1962. Anim. Breed. Abstr. 30 447

Turton, J.D. 1969. The effect of castration on meat production from cattle, sheep and pigs. In: Meat production from entire male animals. p. 1-50. (Ed. D.N. Rhodes). J & A Churchill, London

STORAGE FEEDING OF BEEF BULLS

R. Hardy

Rosemaund Experimental Husbandry Farm, Preston Wynne, Hereford, UK.

ABSTRACT

Storage feeding of grass silage has given a high level of animal performance throughout with a low level of compound supplementation and has offered a potential improvement in pasture utilisation compared to grazing. Successful operation of the system is very dependent on the conservation of high yields of high quality forage, and on the availability of suitable buildings and equipment.

INTRODUCTION

Yields from Italian ryegrass and perennial ryegrass/white clover leys cut three times annually frequently approach 15 t dry matter/ha at Rosemaund. Efficient utilisation of this production with young grazing cattle on the silty soils in Herefordshire is difficult and better utilisation may be achieved by cutting and ensiling the grass. Animal performance may also be improved compared to grazing since checks to animal growth rate caused by diet changes, weather conditions and internal parasites are avoided. Moreover the superior growth potential of the bull compared to the steer can be realised with fewer managerial problems by housing the cattle throughout their lives.

Since August 1979, Rosemaund EHF has been operating a storage feeding system of indoor beef production from young bulls, fed high quality grass silage to appetite with low levels of compound supplement throughout their lives. To date, some 250 animals have been finished in this manner. The results from various breed types, from bulls and hormonal-implanted castrates, and the effects of slaughter weight and age at slaughter are described.

METHOD

Good quality 2 week old calves weighing 50-60 kg were purchased in the open market and reared on a conventional early weaning system, weaning around 5 weeks after arrival on the farm. Two to four weeks later rolled barley with 5-6 per cent of white fishmeal and minerals was introduced and gradually replaced the early weaning compound over the following 2-3 weeks. Hay was available to the calves and grass silage was introduced after 8-10 weeks on the farm and was fed once daily to appetite. At 12-14 weeks (around 120 kg live weight) the barley/fishmeal compound was restricted to 2 kg/head/day. It was fed at this level until slaughter if liveweight gains of at least 1 kg/head/day were being achieved. If lower gains were consistently apparent, the level of compound feed was raised to 4 kg/head/day. Half the bulls in each group were fed at 4 kg/head/day from 40 weeks of age.

On occasions, calves reared off the farm were purchased at 12 weeks of age. These animals were fed silage immediately on arrival along with the barley/fishmeal compound ad libitum initially, and reduced to 2 kg/head/day over the next 2-3 weeks. All the animals referred to were entire males, with the exception of one trial with hormone implanted steers.

RESULTS

Hereford x Friesian Bulls

The results from three batches of 19-24 bulls from 10/11 weeks when compound feed was restricted, were as follows.

TABLE 1   Live and carcass weights (kg) and food consumed (kg/head)
            for three batches of cattle.

	August 1979	August 1980	October 1980
Slaughter weight	407	426	443
Days, arrival (2 weeks old) to slaughter	368	349	396
Daily liveweight gain 10/11 weeks to slaughter	1.01	1.14	1.05
Carcass weight	221	231	243
Food intake from 10/11 weeks:			
Compound (fresh)	720	570	840
Silage DM	920	950	1240
Estimated 'D' value of silage	64	65	65 then 57

For each batch, bulls were split into two groups approximately 40 weeks after arrival; one half continued at 2 kg compound per day until slaughter, the other half was increased to 4 kg.

Bulls of the first two batches were fed high quality silage of about 25% dry matter with 119-130 g/kg DCP and an estimated 'D' value of 64-65. The third batch received more mature silage from 44 weeks with dry matter of 21%, 87 g/kg DCP and in vivo 'D' value of 57. This mature less digestible silage gave poorer bull performance, and in order to maintain 1 kg/head/day liveweight gain 4 kg of compound/head/day were required in the later stages. Despite the increase in compound feeding, it was necessary to keep the bulls for a further 4 weeks to achieve the necessary finish, with an extra input of 0.25 t of silage DM and approximately 200 kg of compound per animal, although these bulls were heavier at slaughter.

Recorded gains of the three batches during the finishing period (from 40 weeks of age) at the two levels of compound feeding are given in Table 2

TABLE 2 Daily gains of cattle (kg)

	Concentrates kg/d		S.E. Diff.
Batch	2 kg	4 kg	
August 1979	1.08	1.41	±0.083
August 1980	1.17	1.38	±0.056
October 1980	0.72	0.97	±0.044

The higher level of compound always increased daily gain but the generally lower performance of the October batch is clearly evident.

British Friesian Bulls

Results in 1981-83 from 44 British Friesian bulls compared with the Hereford x Friesian bulls indicate the following main differences:- time to slaughter, + 12 days; live weight at slaughter, + 23 kg; carcass weight, + 9 kg; compound fed, + 45 kg; silage DM fed, + 110 kg.   EEC carcass external fatness and conformation scores were lower from the Friesians.

Implanted Steers

In 1982, the performance of British Friesian steers implanted with oestradiol 17B at 4½ months of age was compared with bulls. Half of the steers received a further implant of trenbolone acetate 100 days before slaughter. There were 14 animals in each of the 3 groups and they were fed high quality silage throughout (estimated 'D' = 67).

The mean results were as follows:

TABLE 3   Comparative performance of bulls and implanted steers

	Bulls	Implanted steers	S.E. Diff.
Weight at slaughter (kg)	454	430	±4.81
Days 4½ months to slaughter	281	260	±5.23
DLWG (kg)	1.13	1.14	±0.032
Cold carcass weight (kg)	246	231	±3.07
Food intake (kg):			
Compound (fresh)	626	560	−
Silage (DM) t	1.19	1.14	−

Gains were similar for bulls and implanted steers, but the steers matured earlier and were lighter at slaughter. They ate 66 kg/head of compound and 50 kg/head silage dry matter less than the bulls. Resultant financial margins were lower from the steers but their less aggressive nature made on-farm management easier.

Stocking Rates

At Rosemaund, the average yield of silage from two cuts only has been approximately 8 t DM/ha. Silage consumptions of 1-1.25 t DM/head have therefore given grass stocking rates of 7-8 finished cattle/ha. If three or four cuts were taken yields of 12-14 t DM/ha would be attainable, giving potential stocking rates of around 12 cattle/ha.

Effect of Time to Slaughter and Breed Type

During 1982/83, 3 breed types each of 20 animals were assessed. They were early maturing Hereford x Friesian, British Friesian and later maturing Charolais x Friesian. Each group was slaughtered: Early − as soon as external fatness cover was assessed to be 3 to 4 L on the EEC scale, or   Late − 20% heavier than the early group. Very high quality silage was offered throughout (estimated 'D' = 68).

Interim results were as follows:

TABLE 4   Comparative performance of three cattle types (kg/head)

Early slaughter group

	Hereford x Friesian	Friesian	Charolais x Friesian
Weight at start 25.5.82	172	171	142
Weight at slaughter	393	427	429
Days to slaughter	200	227	242
Carcass weight	218.5	233.5	246.1
DLWG	1.11	1.13	1.19
Food intake:			
Compound (fresh)	400	454	484
Silage DM	865	1040	1025

Late slaughter group

	Hereford x Friesian	Friesian	Charolais x Friesian
Weight at start 25.5.82	181	172	145
Weight at slaughter	473	500	514
Days to slaughter	307	300	315
Carcass weight	275.0	282.3	294.5
DLWG	0.95	1.09	1.17
Food intake:			
Compound (fresh)	614	600	630
Silage DM	1360	1450	1430

These results agree with previous U.K. evidence on slaughter weights and gains of a range of breeds and crosses (Allen and Kilkenny, 1980). They also highlight the effect of slaughter weight on food input and overall gain.   In general, they illustrate the wide range of slaughter weights and ages that can be chosen but suggest that the heavier slaughter weight for the Hereford x Friesian was inappropriate since overall gains were sharply reduced.

Financial Margins

Gross margins from the 1979 to 1982 batches have ranged from £530 up to £1,260/ha with an average over five batches of around £1,000/ha. The gross margin analysis includes only the grass growing costs (not total costs of ensilage). These results were assessed from only two ensilage cuts per annum and grass growth from August onwards was available for other stock. Compared with a beef grazing system, there are additional fixed costs for labour, silos, machinery and buildings. Working capital requirement is also high because more beasts per hectare of grass are required than is the case with grazing systems.

REFERENCE
Allen, D. and Kilkenny, J. 1980. Planned beef production. Granada, London.

A COMPARISON OF PROGENY TESTING OF FRIESIAN BULLS INDOORS AND ON PASTURE

H.J. Langholz, M. Suhren and G. Heveling

Institute of Animal Husbandry and Genetics, University of Göttingen,
Albrecht-Thaer-Weg 1, D-3400 Göttingen, Federal German Republic

ABSTRACT

The validity of the standard short term station test for the production systems applied in beef farming was investigated.

The comparison included 9 progeny groups with a total of 326 offspring, which were tested simultaneously on the standard short term test and under farming conditions.

Significant interactions between testing environment and farm environment have been shown, leading to distinct changes in ranking of the sires tested. The magnitude of the interaction increased with increasing differences between the testing environment and the production environment, both regarding fattening intensity and length of fattening period. Interaction in growth parameters was greater than for carcass conformation.These results indicate that the beef testing on stations should be organised to conform as closely as possible to the average fattening environment on farm.

INTRODUCTION

In Northern Germany beef progeny testing has been organised as a short-term test on a concentrate diet, the testing period terminated either by age (300 or 425 days) or by weight (350 or 450 kg). The diet is based on grain and dried sugar beet pulp with some hay.

However, test results have not yet had much impact on breeding decisions. This is partly due to the overwhelming importance of dairy traits in dual-purpose cattle breeding. But in addition there is some distrust of the applicability of the test results to the fattening systems adopted in practice. In bull beef fattening systems in North West Germany both indoors and on pasture much higher final weights are aimed at (Table 1). Since moreover the feeding intensity throughout the systems is lower, depending on the amount and quality of the feeds included, under regular beef farming conditions the fattening periods are longer than the period covered by the test, up to three times in case of finishing from pasture after three grazing periods.

Thus there was a real need to make further comparisons between the standard short term progeny test and progeny testing under beef farming conditions. A first experiment, reported here, consisted of a straight comparison of progeny groups tested simultaneously on station and on selected farms. In a second experiment which is in progress, the short-term station test is compared to a long-term "simulated pasture test" under experimental conditions.

TABLE 1   Bull beef fattening systems in Northern Germany
(traced sample of bulls sold for slaughter in Weser Ems)

Fattening system	No of bulls	Age at slaughter days	Carcass* weight kg	Net* gain g/d	Carcass* grade
I Indoors fattening	187	531	278.5	544	1.42**
II Finishing indoors after 1 grazing period	213	586	290.5	516	1.42
III Finishing indoors after 2 grazing periods	105	765	323.9	433	1.23
IV Finishing from pasture after 2 grazing periods	76	686	289.6	433	1.33
V Finishing from pasture after 3 grazing periods	43	969	342.6	361	0.72

* Least-square means corrected for season of birth and age
** grade E=0, I=1, II=2, III = 3.

Significance of genotype-environmental interactions

In recent years there has been increasing concern about the impact of genotype-environment interactions on breeding decisions especially in ruminant breeding. Experiments on interactions between feeding regimes and fattening performance in cattle have yielded quite different results leading to inconsistent conclusions. Previous studies on the validity of the Northern German short-term progeny test showed no significant interactions with fattening results obtained on farm feeds (Haring et al,1963;Rave, 1973). However the differences in fattening intensity in the systems compared, i.e. sugar beet top silage feeding to 430 kg liveweight and maize silage finishing to 540 days of age, have not been great. On the other hand, in the comprehensive Danish crossbreeding experiment involving a wide range of breed types, genotype-environment interactions were significant at low feeding intensities (Liboriussen et al,1977). Furthermore when testing procedures were extended we observed no, or even a slightly negative, genetic correlation between growth performance in the early and that in the final stage. Krausslich and Averdunk (1973) recorded a genetic correlation between daily gain up to 365 days and daily gain in the period 365-500 days of $r_g = -0.35$ on data from Simmental progeny testing on maize silage. We find similar results for German Friesian performance testing (Jongeling et al,1980). The correlation between daily gain up to one year and daily gain in an 8-week extended period was neutral and significant changes in ranking for growth performance were observed (Table 2). In both studies the variability of growth in the final fattening stages was significantly increased, the coefficient of variation of daily gain in the final fattening stages being about three times as high as that in the early stages.

Thus there is accumulating evidence of genotype-environment interactions in testing for beef performance, with increasing differences in feeding intensities between the testing and the average farm environment and with increasing differences in weight and/or age between termination of test and average conditions in practice.

TABLE 2 Daily gain (g) and rank order ( ) of Friesian bulls before
and after prolongation of performance testing period

Bull	60-365 days	366-426 days
A	1430 (1)	738 (6)
B	1354 (2)	1344 (2)
C	1286 (3)	1501 (1)
D	1256 (4)	1082 (5)
E	1235 (5)	1295 (3)
F	1193 (6)	1295 (4)
G	1177 (7)	574 (7)

These genotype-environment interactions are likely to be related to genetic differences in growth patterns at different stages of tissue growth, especially regarding daily muscle protein retention capacity, and to genetic differences in feed intake, especially with the less concentrated components of the diet.

EXPERIMENTAL COMPARISONS OF SHORT-TERM PROGENY TESTING ON STATION AND
PROGENY TESTING ON FARM

Experimental design and material

Additional progeny were tested under farm conditions from three selected sires in three subsequent test years. For the first team additional testing was done only under pasture conditions but the two other teams were tested also on a maize silage finishing diet.

Fattening on pasture occurs in the typical Northern German 2-year system for autumn-born bulls finished after their second grazing summer. This system includes a more or less restricted feeding regime during the second winter (store period) and concentrate supplement is provided on pasture during the last months of finishing. Three farms were involved in the experiment on which the progeny within sires were randomly distributed.

The maize silage fattening on one farm was of medium intensity compared to the normal standards for that system which allow cattle to reach finished condition at 1½ years of age. Due to the lower dry matter content of maize silage in Northern Germany, 3 kg of concentrates had to be added daily to the ad libitum maize silage intake.

The feeding regime at the test station is based on a full concentrate diet according to weight standards with only small amounts of hay or straw given to prevent rumen disfunction. Increasing amounts of dried sugar beet pulp are given towards the end of the testing period in order to widen the protein : energy ratio.

In Table 3 the experimental design is shown with the total number of offspring in each year and each feeding group, which was finally included

TABLE 3 Experimental design and number of offspring with completed fattening results

		Number of offspring tested		
	Genetic composition of the three	Station	Farm conditions	
Team	Sires	Concentrate feeding to 300 days (365 kg)	Pasture feeding to 735 days (581 kg)	Maize silage feeding to 558 days(562 kg)
1977	50% HF 25% HF DF	29	52	–
1978	100% HF 25% HF DF	29	50	29
1979	100% HF 100% HF DF	33	53	41
	9	91	155	70

% HF = % Holstein Friesian genes; DF = Dutch Friesian

in the statistical analysis. On average each sire was tested by 10.0 offspring on station and by 17.5 on pasture. For the last two teams 12 additional offspring per sire were available for testing on a maize silage fattening diet.

RESULTS

As indicated by the average results obtained on the selected testing regimes (Table 4), field test conditions yielded carcasses which are typical of Northern Germany bull fattening. However while the bulls from pasture tended to be too lean, those fattened on maize silage had already passed beyond the optimum fatness. A level of 4.25% kidney and pelvic fat must be considered to be significantly too fat for German beef market conditions and there was also too much fat cover. Carcasses from the short-term test, weighing 196 kg, on the other hand, were unfinished products in every respect, grading between 2 and 3 on average only. Finally, carcass evaluation by German DLG standards shows the rather inferior quality of these Friesian carcasses which averaged only 30 out of 50 points irrespective of feeding regime.

TABLE 4 Average performance under the different testing regimes (unadjusted data)

Trait	Station test	Field test Finishing on pasture	Field test Maize silage fattening
Final weight (kg)	365.6	580.5	562.1
Age (days)	301	735	556
Daily Gain (g)	1218.9[1]	739.2[2]	957.3[3]
Liveweight gain (g)	1218.6	789.8	1014.2
Net gain (g)	649.7	437.4	569.9
Carcass weight,warm(kg)	196.4	321.5	316.5
Dressing out (%)	54.5	55.4	55.8
Kidney and pelvic fat (%)	1.87	1.89	4.25
Average grade[4]	2.32	1.78	1.87
Fat covering of carcass[5]	2.00	1.74	2.65
Carcass evaluation[6]	30.7	30.9	30.1

[1] 60-301 days of age
[2] 7 to age at slaughter
[3] 7 to age at last regular weighing
[4] E = 1;I = 2;II = 3;III = 4
[5] little = 1;middle = 2;strong = 3
[6] DLG standard,maximum 50 points

Growth and carcass performance data obtained were analysed within test environments in a first series of analyses of variance. Least-squares constants and means for sire effects within years, were computed as main results. The models applied included adjustments for year and age effect. Despite the experimental plan to terminate the test at constant age, small variations in age were unavoidable due to organizational constraints and had to be adjusted for, especially in the pasture test. In the test on pasture additional adjustment was necessary for farm effects and farm x year interaction, since there was a significant difference between years in the fattening pattern within farms.

The following models were applied:

$$Y_{ijkl} = \mu + a_i + b_j + c_{ik} + (a \times b)_{ij} + b_a (A_{ijkl} - \bar{A}) + e_{ijkl} \text{ (pasture)}$$

$$Y_{ikl} = \mu + a_i + c_{ik} + b_a (A_{ikl} - \bar{A}) + e_{ikl} \text{ (maize silage, station test)}$$

where a = year effect

b = farm effect

a x b = effect of farm x year interaction

c = sire effect within year

b_a = linear regression of performance on age at slaughter

A = age at slaughter

The significance of the sire x test environment interaction was studied both by rank correlation between sires in the different test environments and by including sire x test environment interaction in an overall analysis of variance on the year and age corrected data.

Least square sire means for daily gain and net (carcass) gain (Tables 5 and 6) indicate quite distinct differences in the ranking of sires within the different testing environments. The poorest sire in both traits in the short-term station test for example, ranks within the top third of the group under pasture testing and the top sire in maize silage ranks within the poorest group on the station test. Thus, rank correlations were very low (Table 7), while sire x testing environment interaction was highly significant for both growth parameters ($p < 0.01$). However the differences in growth performance between progeny groups became smaller with longer testing periods and decreasing feeding intensity. The difference in net gain between the poorest and the best progeny group was reduced from 64 g on the station test to 37 g on the maize silage test) and 23 g on the pasture test. Maximum group differences in carcass weight at constant age, however, were more or less of the same order, at 19.4, 21.6 and 17.3 kg for station, maize silage and pasture tests, respectively.

TABLE 5 Least-square sire means in daily gain (g)

	Station test[1]	Field test pasture fattening[2]	intensive fattening[3]
$\mu \pm s$	1216 ± 9.31	740 ± 4.34	960 ± 9.52
Sire			
a	1245	750	–
b	1205	752	–
c	1198	717	–
d	1177	738	932
e	1180	731	990
f	1291	751	958
g	1219	729	940
h	1157	741	960
i	1272	750	980

[1] 60–301 days of age; [2] to age of slaughter; [3] to age at last regular weighing

TABLE 6 Least-square sire means in net (carcass) gain (g)

	Station test	Field test pasture fattening	intensive fattening
$\mu \pm s$	651 ± 5.15	437 ± 2.70	570 ± 5.75
Sire			
a	656	446	–
b	630	440	–
c	667	425	–
d	632	432	548
e	633	430	585
f	687	448	577
g	655	430	562
h	623	440	566
i	676	440	581

There were obviously significant differences in growth pattern between progeny groups caused mainly by differences in daily protein retention in the different periods of growth and by differences in feed intake capacity. Highly significant or significant sire x environment interactions for carcass length and fat deposition (Table 8) as well as non-significant rank correlations for these traits underline the differences in growth patterns between progeny groups. Thus a comparison of net gain corrected for constant fat deposition shows the differences in growth pattern more distinctly (Figure 1). Surprisingly differences in carcass quality were not large. Rank correlations indicate a fairly good agreement between station test and field tests in grading and scoring with the strongest relation for front quarter scoring between station and pasture test and for loin and round scoring between the station and maize silage test (Table 10).

For official grading and DLG carcass scoring (Table 9), only a few progeny groups changed their relative position within the various testing environments, as shown by the least-square constants. On the other hand, analyses of variance still showed significant interactions between sire and testing environment for these parameters, especially for official grading. This is due mainly to the highly significant interaction for round scores.

Finally, it should be mentioned that the comparison of the short-term station test with a simulated long-term pasture test on a lower concentrate diet, which is at present in progress leads to similar results.

CONCLUSIONS

The outcome of this experiment clearly confirms the hypothesis that interactions between genetic potential and testing environment can have a significant impact on breeding decisions. There is a strong indication that the testing environment should provide for weights and ages as close as possible to the average fattening environment in the field; thus an ad libitum intake of low-concentrate feed should be allowed corresponding to the nutrient concentration of basic fodder in field fattening. The inclusion of feed intake capacity as a parameter in evaluation and selection is likely to be even more valuable for improving efficiency in dairy production. Therefore the possibility of changing the station test to a computer-controlled ad libitum feeding regime on a low-concentrate pelleted diet should receive special consideration in modern dual-purpose cattle breeding.

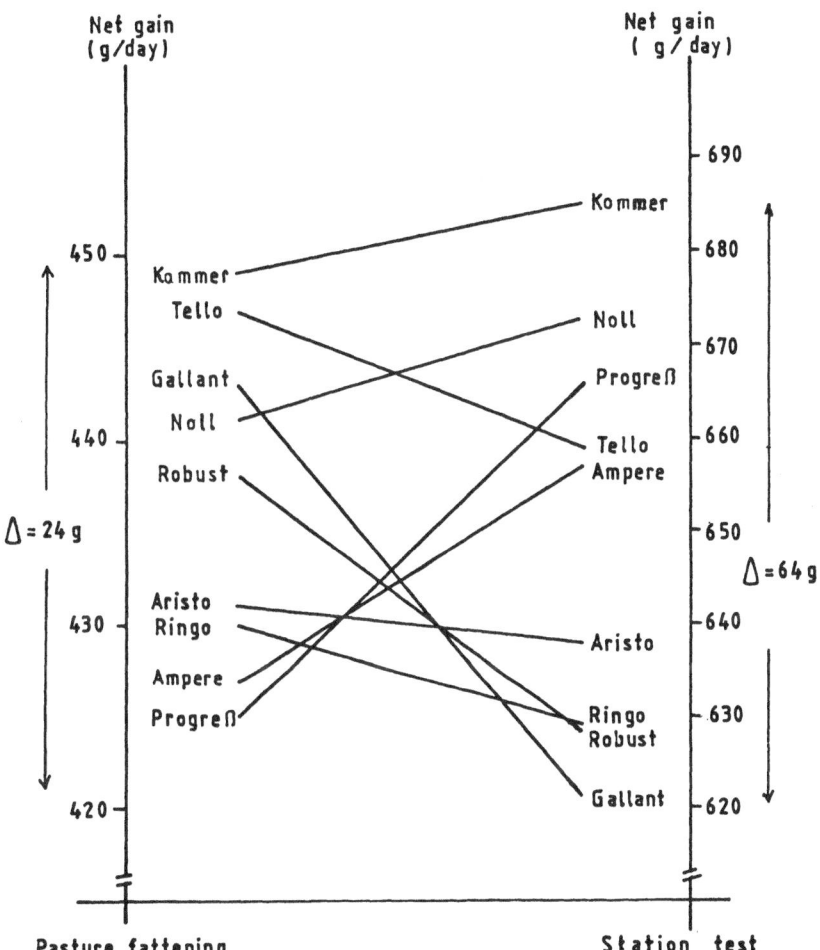

Fig. 1   Net gain adjusted for constant degree of fatness of the individual progeny groups fattened on pasture or tested at station

TABLE 7 Rank correlation between different testing environments in daily gain and net gain

	Pasture test : station test	Maize silage test : station test	Pasture test : maize silage test
Daily gain	.48	.09	.14
Net gain	.10	.37	.20

TABLE 8 Least-square means in percent kidney and pelvic fat

	Station test	Field test Pasture fattening	Intensive fattening
μ ±s	1.87 ± 0.03	1.89 ± 0.04	4.21 ± 0.12
Sire a	2.03	1.83	–
b	1.74	2.00	–
c	1.84	1.85	–
d	2.14	1.93	4.03
e	1.68	1.83	4.21
f	1.80	1.91	4.39
g	1.98	2.08	4.29
h	1.88	1.75	4.41
i	1.75	1.84	3.93

TABLE 9 Least-square sire means in carcass grade[1]

	Station test	Field test Pasture fattening	Intensive fattening
μ ±s	3.30 ± 0.05	2.67 ± 0.42	2.66 ± 0.06
Sire a	3.47	2.48	–
b	3.21	2.76	–
c	3.21	2.77	–
d	3.88	3.02	3.00
e	3.06	2.54	2.46
f	2.96	2.45	2.52
g	3.48	2.81	2.67
h	3.47	2.80	2.89
i	2.95	2.40	2.42

[1]E = 1; I = 2; II = 3; III = 4

TABLE 10   Rank correlation between station and field tests in selected
           parameters of carcass performance

	Coefficient of correlation between:	
	Pasture test : station test	Maize silage test : station test
% kidney and pelvic fat	.05	−.05
DLG judging		
meatiness front quarter	.78 ***	.54
meatiness loin	.68	1.00 ***
meatiness round	.50	.94 **
fat covering	−.70 **	−.26
sum of scores	.60	.83
carcass grade	.90 ***	.94 **

REFERENCES

Haring, F., Weniger, J.H., Gruhn,R. and H.J.Langholz. 1963.   Einsatz von
    Saftfutter und Trockenfutter in der Mast von Jungbullen. Ein Beitrag
    zur   Methodik   der   Nachkommenprüfung   auf   Mastleistung   und
    Schlachtwertbeim Rind. Züchtungskunde **35** 97-113
Jongeling, C.,Goudschaal,H. and Langholz,H.J. 1980. Performance testing of
    Friesian   bulls   for   growth   rate   with   special   reference   to
    short-periodtesting. Polykopie. EVT-Tagung, 1 1, Munchen
Kräusslich,   H.   and   Averdunk,   G.   1973.   Ergebnisse   von
    genetisch-statistischen   Analysen   mit   dem   Datenmaterial   der
    Mast-undSchlachtleistungsprüfungs-anstalten beim Rind in Bayern.
    Polykopie, DGfZ/Gft-Tagung, Gießen
Liboriussen,T.,Neimann-Sørensen and Bech Andersen,B. 1977.   Genotype x
    environment interaction in beef production. In: Proceedings of CEC
    seminar   on   "Crossbreeding   experiments   and   strategy   of   breed
    utilization to increase beef production - EUR **5492e** ,427 - 444
Rave, G. 1973. Genotype-Umwelt-Interaktionen für zwei Prüfungsmethodender
    Nachkommenprüfung auf Fleischleistung beim Rind.
    Züchtungskunde **45** 22-30

SOME CONSIDERATIONS ON PERFORMANCE TESTING ON PASTURE
FOR EUROPEAN BEEF BREEDS

F. Menissier*, C. Béranger** and G. Renand*

* Station de Génétique quantitative et appliquée, Centre National de
  Recherches Zootechniques - INRA, 78350 Jouy-en-Josas,France
** Laboratoire de production de viande bovine, Centre de Recherches
  Zootechnique et Vétérinaire de Theix -INRA, 63122 Ceyrat,Beaumont,France

ABSTRACT

Breed differences in meat production capacity on pasture are partly
due to the selection applied, more or less deliberately, in different beef
production systems. Feed intake, earliness of maturity, muscle growth
capacity and grazing ability could have been changed by these selections.
Since there is enough genetic variability in these traits, improvement of
growth capacity on pasture can be achieved by selection as shown by New
Zealand results. However these results question the validity of central
performance testing on pasture. Moreover selection may increase cow size
and lower their reproductive ability. In France today, selection to
improve beef production is confounded with different production systems (on
pasture, in feedlot), different reproduction systems (AI,natural service)
and with different testing procedures (performance or progeny testing, on
farm or in station). Further joint research efforts between countries and
disciplines would provide a better definition of such responses in
different conditions.

INTRODUCTION

Performance testing is normally carried out on intensively fed young
bulls in barns to ensure the most standardised conditions and to measure
feed intake. Intensive bull beef production provides only 13 to 17% of
French beef production. As Micol and Beranger (1983) show in this volume,
two-year old bulls,steers and heifers are mainly produced on grass, with
two or three grazing periods during their life. The same authors observed
large differences between breeds, such as Normand and Limousin, in growth
rate at pasture for animals reared under the same conditions (Table 1).
Fed indoors, Limousin bulls or steers have the same gain and a better feed
efficiency than Normand. On pasture, Limousin cattle grew 19% less than
Normand and they recovered only during the next winter indoors. These data
show clearly that differences between genotypes are not similar under
grazing or indoor feeding conditions. Therefore genotypic differences
depend largely upon type of production (Frebling et al, 1982). Selection
may however differ according to utilisation of animals. The main
characteristics to be selected for in cattle principally fed on pasture
should be further investigated. Indeed, differences observed between

Limousin and Normand breeds may have arisen indirectly due to selection for different purposes. The Limousin was selected for draft and meat in hilly areas while the Normand was selected for milk and meat in lowland areas more suited to growth and fattening under grazing conditions.

MAIN GENETIC GOALS FOR IMPROVED BEEF PRODUCTION FROM GRASS

At pasture or indoors, animal gain is related to muscle growth capacity which is always the main objective in selection for beef production. But growth rate is dependent on the food intake capacity of the animal, since cattle are fed mainly on grass. Grass intake in turn depends not only on feed intake capacity, but also on the animal's grazing ability. Genotype differences in feed intake capacity are known: Béranger and Micol (1980) pointed out differences between Holstein and Normand bulls and between Maine-Anjou, Charolais and Limousin bulls. Limousin bulls had a rather low feed intake capacity and this could explain their low growth rate at pasture. Along this same line, Micol (1983 - personal communication) observed that on a grass silage diet, Charolais bulls had a lower intake than Holstein and therefore lower gain, in spite of their higher growth potential. Intake capacity could be a limiting factor. Therefore, selection based on feed intake capacity could achieve a better growth rate in grazing animals with high muscular growth potential. Genotype differences in grazing ability are difficult to assess owing to lack of accurate measurement; they could be observed mainly in poor grazing conditions.

If animals are to be fattened at pasture, genotype differences in fat deposition rate become important. In intensive feeding systems with high concentrate diets, animals with low fat deposition and high muscular growth are the most efficient. An adequate level of fatness may be obtained by increasing the dietary energy concentration. But when fed grass, the best animals such as Charolais or Limousin do not reach a high enough level of fatness. Early-maturing animals such as Hereford and Angus are well-known for their ability to be fattened at pasture, at 18-24 months of age. Friesian and Normand steers are easily fattened at pasture, but a large proportion of Limousin or Charolais steers of the same age fail to fatten under the same conditions. In animals such as double-muscled Charolais where the capacity for feed intake and fat deposition is low, grass fattening is very difficult.

At pasture, energy intake could be insufficient as energy concentration of forage is sometimes too low and energy expenditure on grazing is high. Therefore selection for low fat deposition and late maturity, which generally increases the amount and efficiency of meat production, may not be so suitable for beef production on grass. A minimum level of fatness has to be achieved. Selection based on feed efficiency is also of interest for beef production from grass, provided that the capacity for feed intake and fattening are not restricted by this method of selection. As feed efficiency is mainly related to those two characters, such consequences may occur.

Other characters seem important for grazing conditions; hardiness; adaptation to soil, climatic conditions and type of sward; walking ability; resistance to different kinds of parasites etc. Genetic variations and the heritability of such characters are not understood. Breeds or animals selected in a given area are generally well adapted to the environmental conditions. Hardy breeds are especially suitable under difficult conditions. But many breeds like Friesian, Holstein, Charolais or Hereford have displayed great adaptability to various grazing and climatic conditions. It would be interesting to determine some precise biological characters related to these different aptitudes which could be selected efficiently.

POSSIBILITIES AND LIMITS OF SELECTION TOWARD BEEF PRODUCTION FROM GRASSLAND

As performance differences observed between individuals or breeds under grazing conditions are partly induced by a more or less conscious selection of animals for given environmental conditions, the importance of intra-breed genetic variability should be estimated and its possible utilisation in selection programmes considered.

Genetic parameters of cattle growth at pasture

Very few data are available on parameters estimated from grazing animal performance. in the available literature from USA, New Zealand (British breeds at pasture) and France (Charolais), the data summarised in Table 2 point out the following:

a. Heritability of growth characteristics recorded in grazing conditions varies from 0.30 to 0.40, a slightly lower value than that obtained in feed-lot conditions. Reduction of additive genetic variance seems less important under grazing conditions than phenotypic variance, especially for growth rate (Petty and Cartwright,1966). A part of genetic variability is probably not additive under grazing conditions, due to variations in hardiness, grazing capacity and compensatory growth. Final weight seems more heritable than growth rate during the fattening period, although these two characters are correlated (Table 3). For this reason in New Zealand, with early weaning, selection based on final weight (or adjusted for age) seems more efficient for growth improvement than selection based on growth rate (Carter, 1971; Baker et al.,1975)

b. Under grazing or feed-lot conditions, growth rates before and after weaning, weaning weight and final weight are all closely associated. However, postweaning gain is less correlated with weaning weight than weight at one year of age, especially under pasture conditions where phenotypic correlations are negative. Some compensatory growth probably occurs and this type of relation between pre- and post-weaning growth creates difficulties in selection for growth, particularly in performance testing (Dalton and Morris, 1978)

c. There are apparently no estimates of genetic parameters involving factors determining growth at pasture such as feed intake capacity, grazing ability and composition of gain.

The expression of additive genetic variance of growth in beef production systems from grassland depends on good control of environmental conditions. It could be even greater with higher levels of gain. Although it appears lower at pasture than in intensive feeding systems, the genetic variance is sufficient to consider selection for growth under grassland conditions.

Beef selection realised in grazing conditions

Many trials in New Zealand over the past 15 years have clearly shown that growth potential could be improved by selection under grazing conditions (Brumby et al.1963; Carter,1971; Baker et al.1975). Large differences between the progeny of different bulls were noticed for the following: grazing male and female weaning weight, post-weaning growth and liveweight at 14-15 months of age. Progeny testing can be efficiently carried out on pasture with grazing groups of cattle, to improve growth potential, especially when criteria such as the adjusted weight at one year corrected by weaning weight (Baker et al,1975) are used. More recently, as in other countries (USA, Canada, Australia, France) New Zealand workers found progeny testing practicable directly on herds, on farms, using a system of comparison between herds by artificial insemination of some cows with reference bulls (Everitt et al.1976)

Performance testing should also be practicable in grazing conditions and intra-herd. Baker and Carter (1976) noted in comparison with traditional farmer selection, an increment of growth and liveweight at a given age (+4 to 9 kg at weaning, +6 to 19 kg of carcass at 20 months), when they chose sires according to their liveweight at 14 or 20 months under grazing conditions. They also observed similar ranking of sires according to their performance test and progeny test in such conditions (rank correlation :+ 0.4 to +0.8, Baker et al.1975)

Selection experiments in progress (Baker et al 1980) seem to confirm these assessments after the first seven years of intra-herd selection of Angus and Hereford breeds. Compared with the control herd, selection based on liveweight at 13 months of age led to a significant increase in growth and cow weight at first calving. Similarly in Australia, Barlow (1979) selecting bulls on liveweight at one year of age, observed a positive response in progeny yearling weight as early as at the first generation (+18.6 kg between lines selected for and against yearling weight)

DISCUSSION ON PERFORMANCE TESTING PROBLEMS

As noted, individual performance testing of bulls is an efficient and simple means of selection for growth potential and meat production capacity. This individual testing can be carried out in a station with animals from different herds or on farms for intra-herd comparison. In both cases, animals can be reared at pasture or indoors during the testing period.

Individual testing indoors in a station ensures the most standardised conditions and is the most developed system of performance testing in beef breeds (Frebling et al 1972; Lewis and Allen, 1974; Marlowe, 1982) and in dairy and dual purpose breeds (Krausslich, 1974; Bonaiti and Beranger, 1980; Andersen et al,1981). In these conditions and for production of intensive beef fattened indoors, the results of selection through performance testing stations are generally as good as expected in dairy and dual purpose breeds (Averdunk et al.1980; Renand,1983). It is more difficult to assess the efficiency of performance testing in beef breeds. Only a few data correlate performance testing and progeny testing results (Frebling et al,1972;Gaillard et al,1974;Smith et al,1979;Lusweti and Curran,1981;Lopez and Menchaca,1982). In New Zealand,on the basis of the results obtained under grazing conditions , central performance testing stations were established in pasture conditions. In these situations, the first results obtained on the efficiency of this system (Wickham, 1977; Dalton and Morris, 1978; Baker et al,1982) challenge its validity compared with performance testing on farms at pasture (Carter, 1971; Baker et al,1975). With more than 66 proven sires, the correlation was three times less than expected (+0.15 versus +0.48) betwen the final liveweight of proven bulls and the final liveweight of their progeny recorded in station (crossbreed with dairy breed). Therefore, the realised heritability of final weight is very low (0.06±0.06) compared with the value generally observed in indoor feeding performance testing stations (0.30 to 0.70).

These results indicate that there are some limits to the efficiency of performance testing in central stations, especially under grazing conditions (Dalton and Morris, 1978). In performance testing stations, even with indoor feeding, one of the main problems is the influence of previous growth and rearing conditions on performance during the testing period. Growth rate and final weight correlate more or less with initial weight and previous growth rate (Preston and Willis, 1970; Lewis and Allen, 1974; Dutertre, 1975; Dalton, 1976; Morris, 1981; Renand, 1983). Initial and final weight are frequently well correlated (+0.4 to +0.9), so many people recommend only the growth rate in station as a criterion of selection, rather than final weight. However, some compensatory growth may occur and this can be more frequent under grazing conditions. This phenomenon can induce negative environmental correlations between pre-and post-weaning growth. On the other hand, positive genetic correlations should occur between previous and actual growth in relation to the individual growth potential of each animal (Table 3). This parameter includes the genetic effect of herd of origin and makes it difficult to correct this factor.

To reduce the effect of previous feeding and management of bulls, some proposals have been made (Lewis and Allen, 1974; Krausslich, 1974; Richardson, 1979; Bonaiti and Beranger, 1980; Andersen et al,1981; Okantah

and Curran, 1982; Patterson et al,1982; Renand, 1983). These include:
(a) Starting the test at an earlier age. This is difficult in suckler cow herds, but is suitable for Charolais in Cuba or for the Blonde d'Aquitaine for veal production in France (b) Increasing the length of the test period (4 to 5 months) with a longer period of adaptation. This does not appear to be sufficient under grazing conditions (Dalton and Morris, 1978).
(c) Elimination of extreme animals by instituting minimum and maximum initial weights (d) Provision of high feeding levels, not taking animal weight into account (e) Criteria for selection correctly combined into an index of selection, e.g. growth rate, final weight adjusted for age, growth rate corrected according to initial weight.

If the herd size is large enough and the selection conducted within the herd, it is obvious that performance testing in farms is as efficient as in stations because of the decrease in the effect of previous conditions. This is the present assumption in New Zealand (Baker et al,1982). But in Western Europe, herd size is too small for that purpose. With the Hereford breed under British conditions, Smith et al (1979) found that selection was more efficient in performance testing stations than on farms. Apparently, the figures from Lusweti and Curran (1982) did not confirm this efficiency. On-farm testing allows a wider basis for selection. If performance testing is carried out indoors, it may be possible to take feed intake capacity into account (Bonaiti and Beranger, 1980; Andersen et al, 1981) (Table 4).

As shown in this review, the question of performance testing is still unsettled and needs more research. It is difficult to carry out work indoors, and even more difficult at pasture, both theoretically and practically. It is also necessary to bear in mind that the improvement of size and fleshiness of cattle could induce a negative effect on dam maternal qualities (Menissier, 1976). In the Charolais breed, with heifers station-tested under grazing conditions, negative genetic correlations have been found between weight and conformation at 18 months of age, and fertility (-0.25 and -0.41 respectively) and calving ability (-0.21 and -0.51 respectively). The consequences of selection for growth rate on calving ability are now better known (Menissier et al,1981). If preliminary results obtained in New Zealand and in Australia with British breeds do not show a negative effect on fertility and calving ability (birth weight/pelvic opening) from selection for increased size and weight of heifers or cows (Barlow, 1979; Morris and Baker, 1982), similar selection experiments should be conducted on continental beef breeds in Europe.

PRESENT SITUATION OF PERFORMANCE TESTING IN BEEF CATTLE IN FRANCE

Selection is carried out conventionally by breeders and by artificial insemination units (Beranger and Menissier, 1981; Menissier et al, 1982). AI bull selection, which was primarily directed toward muscle development for crossbreeding with dairy or dual purpose cattle, now takes into account reproductive performance of the female measured by progeny testing in station. Moreover in order to give more importance to selection of breeding animals for natural mating an adapted progeny and performance test has been developed. There are now several situations that take into account some of the variations in French beef production systems (Table 5)

Selection of AI bulls for terminal crossing

Performance testing in stations is important and appears to be efficient, particularly after some recent adjustments (Gaillard et al, 1974,1982; Dutertre, 1975; Bonaiti and Beranger, 1980). As animals are used in crossbreeding with dairy breeds which are generally early-maturing and with high feed intake capacity, the main goals of selection are muscular growth potential related to growth rate, conformation, body composition and feed efficiency. Therefore animals are fed a pelleted diet, according to their liveweight, to reach high growth levels after two months of adaptation on a moderate level of gain. The selection index used for ranking animals combines growth (liveweight adjusted by age and test daily gain), fleshiness and feed efficiency and seems to give good results (Renand, 1983).

Selection of AI bulls for pure breeding

Feed intake capacity should be important in selection with respect to the main feeding systems, namely, beef production from grassland and beef cows fed mainly on roughages. These traits are not directly estimated in the performance tests which are conducted as in the stations for crossbreeding purposes noted above (with some differences in weight of characters). A large part of this type of selection is thought to be achieved by selection of the bull's dam plus the bull's progeny test on a daughter reared at pasture in stations (18-month weight related to grazing performance). These systems should perhaps be reconsidered for some breeds like Limousin or Blonde d'Aquitaine which have low feed intake capacities. In the Charolais breed, the problem is perhaps less acute and some performance testing is carried out on 2-year old bulls fed a roughage diet. Weight at 2 years could be an efficient criterion for selecting bulls according to size and feed intake capacity.

Selection of bulls for natural service in specialised beef breeds

This selection is very important, as 40 to 80% of cows are mated to bulls on the farm (Menissier et al,1982). As the herd size is generally small, the best system seems to be progeny testing on the farm, by utilising a reference AI sire on some cows over several herds to connect them together (Foulley and Sapa, 1982). This has started to be developed in Limousin and Charolais herds. However the number of tested bulls still remains too small. Performance testing in stations is also being developed to produce bulls for natural mating. Bulls are fed with hay ad libitum and a given amount of concentrates. The objective is to select animals for pure breeding according to their muscle growth potential, feed intake capacity and conformation. These stations could be local, or national to compare all the best animals of the breeds from different areas.

Selection of bulls in hardy breeds for beef production

In hardy breeds, selection for muscle growth potential and feed intake is carried out at performance testing stations which supply bulls for natural mating and also for AI. Since performance testing on farms is difficult, these stations which are managed as the above stations for beef breed natural service, have been set up in the hardy breed areas (Salers, Aubrac, Gasconne)

Hence the present situation in France is a compromise between the diversity of French production systems, types of sire utilisation, and possibilities of the different methods of selection.

CONCLUSIONS

It is obvious that performance testing could be organised according to the various ways which more or less take into account beef production in grasslands. But there is no experimental evidence of the different efficiencies of these different ways. Further investigation is needed along with more experimentation on this complicated subject. Research should be developed on the importance of selection for feed intake capacity in relation to the selection goals in the different breeds and on the consequences of such a selection in the different production systems. Such research will require many animals and considerable facilities. This could most effectively be done in a common project involving several different countries, as in an EEC programme.

But it is necessary to bear in mind that the different beef production systems can themselves be adapted to different breeds. For example, to fatten late maturing animals at pasture, steer production might be preferable. Alternatively anabolic agents could be used for early-maturing animals. Compromise in selection is possible to a certain extent, but could restrain genetic progress too much. As selection programmes are generally expensive and difficult to organise, some main directions which are the most efficient will have to be chosen.

REFERENCES

Andersen, B.B., De Baerdemaeker, A.,Bittante,G.,Bonaiti,B.,Colleau,J.J., Fimland, E., Jansen, J.,Lewis, W.H.E., Politiek,R.D., Seeland, G., Teehan, T.J., Werkmeister, F. 1981. Performance testing on bulls in AI: report of a working group of the Commission on cattle production. Livest.prod.Sci., 8 101-119

Averdunk, G., Alps, H. Gottschalk, A.,Fusseder,J. 1980. Relationship between performance test traits of the sire and fattening and carcass traits of his progenies. 31st Annual meeting, EAAP, 1-4th September,1980, München (RFA), 9p

Baker, R.L., Carter,A.H. 1976. The value of on-farm performance selection of Angus and Hereford bulls. Proc. NZ Soc. Anim. Prod. 36 216-221

Baker, R.L., Carter,A.H., Beatson,P.R. 1975. Progeny testing Angus and Hereford bulls for growth performance. Proc. NZ Soc Anim.Prod. 35 103-111

Baker,R.L., Carter, A.H., Hunter, J.C. 1980. Preliminary results of selection for yearling or 18-month weight in Angus and Hereford cattle. Proc. NZ Soc.Anim.Prod. 40 304-311

Baker, R.L.,Wickham,B.W., Morris,C.A. 1982. The accuracy of central bull performance tests in New Zealand as evaluated by subsequent progeny testing. 2nd World Congress on genetics applied to livestock production, 4-8th October 1982, Madrid (SP), 8 300-304

Barlow, R. 1979. Short term responses to selection for high and low yearling gain in Angus cattle. Proc. Symposium on "Selection experiments in Laboratory and Domestic animals", 21-22 July,1979, Harrogate (UK), 144-146

Beranger, C. Menissier,F. 1981. Les races bovines allaitantes. Rapport de la Commission des Recherches bovines de l'INRA. Bull.tech.du CRVZ de Theix, Inst.nat.Rech.agr.Fr., 43 5-14

Beranger, C., Micol,D. 1980. Intake in relation to the animal. Ann.Zootech., 29 (spec.issue),209-226

Bonaiti,B., Béranger, C. 1980. Some considerations about performance testing of beef cattle in France. 31st Annual Meeting EAAP, 1-4th September, 1980, München (RFA),7p

Brumby,P.J., Walker, D.E.K. and Gallagher, R.M. 1963. Factors associated with growth in beef cattle. NZ. J. agric. Res. 6 526-537

Carter, A.H. 1971. Effectiveness of growth performance selection in cattle. Proc. NZ Soc.Anim.Prod., 31 151-163

Dalton,D.C. 1976. An analysis of Angus Central bull performance tests in New Zealand. Proc. NZ Soc.Anim.Prod. 36 211-215

Dalton,D.C,Morris,C.A. 1978. A review of Central performance testing of beef bulls and of recent research in New Zealand. Livest.Prod.Sci. 5 147-157

Dutertre,M. 1975. Modalités d'application,bilan et analyse du contrôle individuel des taureaux utilisés en insémination artificielle. Mémoire de fin d'études,ISA de Beauvais (unpublished)

Everitt,G.C., Jury, K.E, Ward, J.D.B.1976. On-farm progeny testing for beef production. Proc. NZ Soc.Anim.Prod. 36 222-230

Foulley,J.L.,Sapa,J. 1982. The French evaluation program for natural service bulls using AI sire progeny as herd ties. Winter Conf.1982. Ed. British Cattle Breeders Club (Digest 37), 64-68

Frebling,J. Gaillard,J.,Vissac,B. 1972. Mise en place et efficacité du schéma de sélection des taureaux de races à viande pour le croisement industriel. Bull.tech.Dept.Génét. anim.,INRA Fr., 15 23-55

Frebling,J. Bonaiti,B., Bibe,B.,Gillard,P.,Menissier,F.,Renand,G. 1982. Comparison of fattening and slaughter performances between Charolais, Limousin, Maine-Anjou and Hereford breeds according to various production types. 2nd World Congress on genetics applied to livestock production, 4-8th October,1980, Madrid (SP), 3 334-339

Gaillard,J.,Foulley,J.L., Menissier,F. 1974. Observations sur l'efficacité du choix sur ascendance paternelle et performances individuelles des taureaux de races à viande destinés au croisement terminal. 1st World Congress on genetics applied to livestock production, 7-11th October,1974, Madrid (SP), 3 877-887

Gaillard,J., Foulley,J.L., Renand,G., Menissier,F. 1982. Limits of on-the farm progeny testing of crossbred calves commercialised shortly after birth, for beef sire evaluation. 2nd World Congress on genetics applied to livestock production, 4-8th October 1980, Madrid (SP), 8 346-350

Koch,R.M., Gregory,K.E., Cundiff,L.V. 1982. Critical analysis of selection methods and experiments in beef cattle and consequences upon selection programs applied. 2nd World Congress on genetics applied to livestock production, 4-8th October 1982, Madrid (SP), 5 514-526

Krausslich,H. 1974. General recommendations on procedures for performance progeny testing for beef characteristics. Livest. Prod. Sci. 1 33-45

Lewis,W.H.E.,Allen,D.M. 1974. Performance testing for beef characteristics. 1st World Congress on genetics applied to livestock production, 7-11th October 1974, 1 671-679

Lopez,D. Menchaca,M. 1982. A note of the year,season and sire effects on the daily gain of Charolais cattle in performance test stations. Cuban J. Agric. Sci., 16 137-140

Lusweti,E.C.,Curran,M.K. 1981. Estimates of environmental effects and genetic parameters in beef cattle using both farm and station test records. 76th Meeting Brit.Soc.Anim.Prod.1981, Harrogate (UK). Anim.Prod. 32 382 (Abstr.)

Marlowe,T.J. 1982. Development of beef cattle performance testing in the United States. 2nd World Congress on genetics applied to livestock production,4-8th October,1982,Madrid,(SP), **8** 399-404

Menissier, F. 1976. Comments on optimization of cattle breeding schemes: beef breeds for suckling herds. A review. Ann. Génét. Sél. anim., **8** 71-87

Menissier, F., Foulley, J.L., Gogue, J. 1975. Estimation des paramètres génétiques et phénotypiques en race charolaise, pour les génisses vêlant à 2 ans en station de contrôle des qualitiés d'élevage (unpublished)

Menissier, FG.,Foulley,J.L. and Pattie,W.A. 1981. The calving ability of the Charolais breed in France and its possibilities for genetic improvement. Irish Vet. J. **35** 128-134

Menissier, F., Foulley, J.L., Sapa, J. 1982. Selection of French beef breeds for purebreeding. 2nd World Congress on genetics applied to livestock producion, 4-8th October, 1982, Madrid (SP), **8** 314-324

Micol, D. 1982. Production de Jeunes Taureaux - Production de boeufs. In:"Les principaux types de production de viande en race bovine limousine". Bull. tech, CRVZ,Theix, INRA Fr., **48** (spec issue), 65-70,71-75

Morris, C.A. 1981. Herd effects on the growth of beef bulls from different sources tested together under grazing conditions. NZ Journal of Agric. Res., **24** 11-20

Morris,C.A., Baker,R.L. 1982. Cow weights and other correlated responses yearling or 18-month weight selection. 2nd World Congress on genetics applied to livestock production, 4-8th October,1982, Madrid (SP), **8** 294-299

Okantah, S.A., Curran,M.K. 1982. A review of the effects of the environment in the central performance testing of beef cattle. World Rev. Anim.Prod., **18** (2) 39-48

Patterson, T.B., Meadows, G.B., McGuire,J.A. 1982. An analysis of 26 years of beef bull performance testing at Auburn University. Alabama Agric. Exp. Stat.,Auburn Univ. Bull No.536, 15p

Petty, R.R.,Cartwright,T.C. 1966. A summary of genetic and environmental statistics for growth and conformation traits of young beef cattle. Texas ASM University, Dept. tech.report No.5 (January 1966),55p

Preston,T.R., Willis, M.B. 1970. Intensive Beef Production. Ed.Pergamon Press,Oxford,566p.

Renand,G. 1983. Variabilité génétique et sélection des aptitudes bouchères chez les bovins. Thesis (in preparation)

Richardson,F.D. 1979. Some nutritional factors influencing the growth and efficiency of beef cattle at different ages and their implications for the design of regimes for the performance testing of young bulls. A review. Rhod. J. agric. Res., **17** 71-87

Smith,C.,Steane,D.E.,Jordan,C. 1979. Progeny test results on Hereford bulls weight-recorded on the farm. Anim.Prod. **28** 49-53

Wickham, B.W. 1977. The relationships between central test station performance and subsequent progeny performance for growth traits of Hereford bulls. Proc. NZ Soc. Anim.Prod. **37** 89-95

TABLE 1 Comparison between Normand and Limousin cattle at pasture or fed indoors (from Micol, 1982)

GROUP OF CATTLE :	BULLS :				STEERS :	
	Limousin	Normand	Limousin	Normand	Limousin	Normand
Grazing period (between 14 and 20 months) :						
• Duration (day)..........	180	180	192	192	168	168
• Initial weight (kg)......	429	420	405	408	421	408
• Average daily gain (g)......	789	944	763	911	678	848
Indoor fattening :						
• Duration (day)............	91	91	115	112		
• Initial weight (kg)........	590	612	547	581		
• Average daily gain (g/d)......	1561	1418	1192	1234		
• Carcass weight (kg)........	456	431	435	423		
• Feed efficiency (g/FU)......	157	134	135	122		
Fattening at pasture (between 24 and 30 months) :						
• Duration (day)............					122	114
• Initial weight (kg)........					590	599
• Average daily gain (g/d)......					729	938
• Carcass weight (kg)........					409	391

TABLE 2 Heritability of growth estimated on pasture or feedlot conditions (main figures from literature)

AUTHORS	COMMENT	TRAITS: BIRTH WEIGHT	PREWEANING GROWTH	WEANING WEIGHT	WEANING SCORE	POSTWEANING GROWTH	YEARLING WEIGHT	FINAL WEIGHT	FINAL SCORE
FEEDLOT:									
PETTY and CARTWRIGHT (1966)	Bibliography review (b)	(0.44)	(0.31)	(0.28)	(0.32)	0.52	-	0.58	0.36
PRESTON and WILLIS (1970)	Bibliography review (a)	0.38	0.27	0.30	-	0.52	-	-	-
RENAND (1983)	Bibliography review (a)	0.42	-	0.30	-	0.47	0.45		-
RENAND (1983)	Charolais, crossbred bulls, station (FR)	0.32	-	0.18	0.21	0.41	0.32	-	0.21
PASTURE:									
PETTY and CARTWRIGHT (1966)	Bibliography review (b)	(0.44)	(0.31)	(0.28)	(0.32)	0.30	0.41	-	0.22
CARTER (1971)	In test herds (NZ)	-	-	0.25	-	~0	0.40	-	-
BAKER et al. (1975)	In test herds (NZ)	0.28	-	0.20	-	0.20	0.45	-	-
LISWETI and CURRAN (1981)	Field data (UK)	-	-	0.12	-	-	0.20	-	-
MENISSIER et al. (1975)	Charolais, purebred heifers, station (FR)	-	-	0.22	-	0.21	0.33	-	0.48

(a) included some figures on pasture conditions (b) common value on pasture and feedlot conditions before weaning

137

TABLE 3 Phenotypic and genetic correlations between growth traits on pasture or feedlot conditions
(some figures from literature)

GENETIC (or between sire) CORRELATIONS:	(a)	BIRTH WEIGHT: Pasture:	BIRTH WEIGHT: Feedlot:	PREWEANING GROWTH: Pasture:	PREWEANING GROWTH: Feedlot:	WEANING WEIGHT: Pasture:	WEANING WEIGHT: Feedlot:	POSTWEANING GROWTH: Pasture:	POSTWEANING GROWTH: Feedlot:	YEARLING OR FINAL WEIGHT: Pasture:	YEARLING OR FINAL WEIGHT: Feedlot:
BIRTH WEIGHT (b)	NZ1,	−				+ 0.54		− 0.03		+ 0.36	
	NZ2,		−			+ 0.62		+ 0.01		+ 0.45	
	FR1,2		−		+ 0.38		+ 0.58		+ 0.15		+ 0.26
	US1,2		−				+ 0.25		+ 0.56		+ 0.64
PREWEANING GROWTH (b)	NZ1,	+ 0.23		−		+ 0.98					
	NZ2,			−							
	FR1,2		+ 0.23		−		+ 0.98				+ 0.73
	US1,2				−						
WEANING WEIGHT (b)	NZ1,	+ 0.42		+ 0.98		−		+ 0.07		+ 0.75	
	NZ2,							+ 0.17		+ 0.76	
	FR1,2		+ 0.11		+ 0.97		−	+ 0.11	+ 0.54	+ 0.87	+ 0.78
	US1,2		+ 0.39					+ 0.08	+ 0.58	+ 0.67	+ 0.79
POSTWEANING (b)	NZ1,	+ 0.08		− 0.20		− 0.17		−		+ 0.72	
	NZ2,									+ 0.57	
	FR1,2		+ 0.18			− 0.29	− 0.23		−	+ 0.59	+ 0.93
	US1,2		+ 0.30		+ 0.14	+ 0.25	+ 0.17			+ 0.81	+ 0.86
FINAL OR YEARLING WEIGHT (b)	NZ1,	+ 0.40		+ 0.64		+ 0.68		+ 0.60		−	
	NZ2,									−	
	FR1,2		+ 0.18		+ 0.63	+ 0.81	+ 0.64	+ 0.33	+ 0.81	−	
	US1,2		+ 0.42			+ 0.64	+ 0.65	+ 0.63	+ 0.77		

PHENOTYPIC CORRELATIONS

(a) genetic correlations above diagonal, phenotypic correlations below diagonal

(b) NZ1 = Carter (1971); NZ2 = Baker et al (1975); FR1 = purebred Charolais heifers, Menissier et al (1975); FR2 = crossbred Charolais bulls, Renand (1983); US1,2 = bibliography review, Petty and Cartwright (1966)

TABLE 4 Importance of feeding system for selection response and breeding objective (adapted from Andersen et al,1981; Bonaiti and Beranger, 1980)

FEEDING SYSTEM: ROUGHAGE	CONCENTRATE	GROWTH RATE LEVEL	SELECTION TRAITS ON	SELECTION RESPONSE ON: FEED INTAKE CAPACITY	LEAN TISSUE GROWTH CAPACITY	RESIDUAL FEED EFFICIENCY	BREEDING OBJECTIVE
1.Restricted	/ Restricted	low	growth rate	+	++	+++	
Restricted	/ Restricted	high	growth rate	++	+++	+++	Beef from cereals.
2.Restricted	/ Ad libitum	high	growth rate	+++ (for concentrate)	++	++	
3.Ad libitum	/ Restricted	high	growth rate	+++ (for roughage)	+	++	Beef from grass.
4.Ad libitum	/ Ad libitum (complete diet)	high	growth rate and feed efficiency	+++	++	+	

TABLE 5   Main characteristics of performance test station in France for bulls from specialised and hardy beef breeds

SELECTION PROGRAMME OF SIRE :	ABILITY TO BE IMPROVED ON STATION :	MANAGEMENT :				SELECTION : (selection rate)	CAPACITY : (station, bulls)
		TIME (months): Adaptation + control :	GROWTH RATE LEVEL :	DIET :	FEEDING SYSTEM :		
CROSSBREEDING FOR BEEF, by A.I. : (CH, BA, Li)	1.High muscle growth rate, 2.lean body contents, 3.feed efficiency (residual), 4.feed intake capacity (for concentrate).	2 months + 4 months	HIGH (CH>1500, BA>1400, Li>1300, g/day)	COMPLET DIET (60p.100 dehydrated lucern, 30p.100 cereals)	1 month AD LIBITUM and 3 months LIMITED (according to live weight and fixed level growth rate)	.Weight adjusted by age and growth rate on control period. .Beef conformation (fleshiness). .Feed intake adjusted by weight and gain.(p=50 to 20p.100)	CH=4 stat.(40 to 80d/year). BA=1 stat.(40d/year) Li=2 stat.(45d/year)
PUREBREEDING FOR SPECIALISED BEEF BREEDS, by A.I. : (CH,BA,Li)	1.high muscle growth rate, 2.lean body contents, 3.feed efficiency (residual), 4.feed intake capacity (for roughage).	4 months				.Weight adjusted for age and growth rate on control period. .Body score conformation (size, fleshiness) .Feed intake adjusted by weight and gain.(p=20p.100)	CH=1 stat.(40d/year) BA and LI = included in the crossbreeding program.
(only CH)	1.size and growth rate, 2.feed intake capacity (for roughage) 3.high muscle growth rate.	4 months + 3 months	MEDIUM (CH:1300 then 1100g/day)	HAY + CONCENTRATE.	ROUGHAGE AD LIBITUM + RESTRICTED CONCENTRATE (Independent of between bull weight differences)	.Weight adjusted for age. .Body score conformation (size, fleshiness). (p=30p.100)	CH = 1 stat. (30d/year ; plus 20 to 70d in project).
SPECIALIZED BEEF BREEDS, by NATURAL SERVICE : (CH,LI)	1.high muscle growth rate 2.feed intake capacity (for roughage) 3.size	1 month + 4 to 5 Months	HIGH to MEDIUM (CH:1400, Li:1300, then 1200, g/day)	HAY (or mais silage) + CONCENTRATE.	ROUGHAGE AD LIBITUM + RESTRICTED CONCENTRATE (Independent of between bull weight differences).	.Weight adjusted by age and growth rate on control period. .Body score conformation (size, fleshiness).	CH=2 stat.(100 to 150 d/year) Li=2 stat. (250d/year) + 1 stat. (400d, in project.)
HARDY BREEDS FOR BEEF, by NATURAL SERVICE : (SA,AU,GA)	1.feed intake capacity (for roughage) 2.high muscle growth rate, 3.size.		HIGH to MEDIUM (SA=1200, AU=1000, GA=1000, g/day)			.Body score conformation (size, fleshiness). (p:CH and Li:50p. 100;GA:50p.100, AU and SA 60 to 65=p. 100).	SA=1 stat.(40d/year) AU=1 stat.(70d/year) GA=2 stat.(45d/year)

CH=Charolais, BA=Blond d'Aquitaine, Li=Limousin, SA=Salers, AU=Aubrac, GA=Gascon.

MEASUREMENT OF GRAZING BEHAVIOUR AND HERBAGE INTAKE ON TWO
DIFFERENT GRAZING MANAGEMENT SYSTEMS FOR BEEF PRODUCTION

M. O'Sullivan

The Agricultural Institute, Johnstown Castle, Wexford, Ireland

ABSTRACT

Two systems of grazing management for beef production were compared, a continuously grazed system with a 20 x 1 day rotational paddock grazing system at two stocking rates for three years. No difference was obtained in net herbage accumulation between the systems, but the high stocking rate reduced herbage production by 7.5%. Rotational grazing increased animal production per hectare by 33% at the high stocking rate and by 7.6% at the low stocking rate. Although the animals grazed pastures of different digestibilities, they always selected material of similar digestibility. The length of time spent grazing and the distance walked in the process was greater for the continuously grazed animals than for the rotationally grazed animals. Consequently the set stocked cattle had a 44% greater grazing energy expenditure than the rotationally grazed cattle. The efficiency of food conversion was greater under rotational grazing as a result of lower maintenance energy requirements.

INTRODUCTION

The first Irish work on grazing systems was by Drew and Deasy (1937) who reported that rotational grazing by store cattle led to an increase of 27% in production per hectare. In the 1960s, Conway (1962a, 1962b, 1964), in experiments with beef cattle, showed advantages to rotational grazing of between 21 and 91% at high stocking rates. Similar advantages to rotational grazing have been found with dairy cows at high stocking rates (McCarthy, 1979;McMeekan, 1956; McMeekan & Walshe, 1963)

There are however, many reports in the literature showing little or no advantage to rotational grazing. In a review of European work, Ernst et al (1980) summarised nine different trials and concluded that there was an advantage of 1.5% for dairy cows and 6% for beef cattle by grazing a paddock system. Similar results in favour of rotational grazing were also reported by Marsh (1975). The value however, of such appraisals is extremely doubtful. Most experiments show an advantage to rotational grazing when the ratio of herbage produced to the weight of grazing animal is low. This ratio varies widely with fertiliser use, sward type, stocking rate and probably paddock number. In both of the above assessments, all these parameters varied widely from experiment to experiment and consequently it would be surprising if any difference was shown between the two systems of grazing management.

In view of the contradictions in the literature concerning the merits of different systems of grazing, it seems more important to identify the criteria that lead to an advantage of one system over another; only then will it be possible to provide objective grazing guidelines for the farmer. With this objective, detailed measurements of dry matter production, liveweight gain, herbage intake and animal behaviour were made on rotational and continuous systems of grazing for intensive beef production in a three-year experiment.

EXPERIMENTAL

Experimental area

The pasture was sown two years previously with the perennial ryegrass Cropper. An area of 8.36 hectares was allocated between four treatments as follows: continuous grazing and rotational grazing each at a low and a high stocking rate. Stocking rate was controlled by varying the size of the area while keeping animal numbers constant between treatments. At both stocking rates the rotationally grazed area was divided into 20 paddocks, each of which was grazed for a day. 370 kg/ha of 0:7:30 fertilizer were applied in autumn and nitrogen was applied during the grazing season as calcium ammonium nitrate at the rate of 230 kg N/ha in 1978 and 350 kg N/ha in 1979 and 1980.

Allocation of animals

Eighty evenly sized animals were chosen from a group of one hundred that had been overwintered on silage. They were blocked according to weight and randomly allocated from within blocks to the four treatments, with twenty cattle per treatment. Initial weights varied from 190 to 250 kg. All animals were dosed twice during the grazing season to control liver fluke and intestinal parasites. The two stocking rates, which varied slightly from year to year, were approximately 1890 kg/ha for the low and 2740 kg/ha for the high. Reductions were made in stocking rate twice during the year, by taking animals off the experimental area.

Sward measurements

Net herbage accumulation was estimated using quadrats (1.667 x 0.15M) cut to ground level with Sunbeam sheep shears. On the rotationally grazed treatments pre-and post-grazing samples were taken in 10 out of the 20 paddocks. Six pre- and six post-grazed paired quadrats were taken on the low stocking rate and five on the high stocking rate.

Net herbage production was calculated using the formula:

$$\text{Net Production} = Pre_1 + Pre_2 - Post_1 \text{-----} + Pre_n - Post_{n-1}$$

The continuously grazed plots were arbitrarily divided into three areas and one animal exclusion cage placed on each. Three samples were taken from inside the cage and nine from outside. Cages were randomly moved weekly at the start of the season, and then every two weeks as the grass growth rate decreased.

Animal measurements

Animals were weighed every cycle, after fasting for 16 hours. At the end of the 1980 grazing season a number of animals from each treatment were slaughtered to determine carcass weights. Herbage intake was measured according to the method of Hodgson and Rodriguez (1970) once every cycle, from estimates of faecal output using the chromic oxide dilution technique and from the digestibility of herbage selected by oesophageally-fistulated animals. Ten animals per treatment were dosed twice daily with 10 g of chromic oxide impregnated paper for twelve days. Faecal samples were collected twice daily on the last five days of the dosing period and pooled for analysis. Chromium was estimated by atomic absorption according to Williams et al (1962). Four animals fistulated at the oesophagus sampled the four treatment areas before and after grazing, in such a way that each animal sampled the experimental area during the measurement period. Extrusa samples were immediately stored on ice, subsequently freeze-dried and analysed by the standard in-vitro digestibility technique (Tilley and Terry, 1963).

Measurements of animal behaviour were made at intervals throughout 1980. Grazing time was measured by observing the activity of six differently marked animals per treatment, every ten minutes from dawn to dusk. Grazing during darkness was checked using Vibracorders on two animals per treatment. The distance walked during grazing was calculated from traces on a scaled map of the paddock of the actual movement of two animals per treatment during daylight hours.

RESULTS

There was no difference in the average amount of dry matter produced by the two systems of management over the three years. In 1979 the

rotationally grazed treatment produced 14% more dry matter but the reverse
was true in 1980 and the average over the three years showed no significant
difference (Table 1)

TABLE 1 Dry matter production and liveweight gain under continuous
and rotational grazing systems (av 3 years)

	DM production kg/ha	Total LWG kg/ha	Accumulated LWG per average animal kg
Continuous grazing			
LSR	9851	996	143
HSR	9115	940	92
Rotational grazing			
LSR	9997	1072	158
HSR	9244	1252	129
SE mean and significance	219.8*	33.9***	4.07***

Stocking rate had a greater effect on dry matter production than
system of grazing, the high stocking rate causing a reduction of
approximately 7.5% in both continuous and rotational grazing every year.

At the high stocking rate there was an increase of 33% in liveweight
gain per hectare when animals were rotationally grazed rather than set
stocked. At the lower stocking rate the advantage was only 7.6% and one
would expect that if the stocking rate was reduced still further, no
difference would be obtained between the two systems. The effect of
stocking rate varied with the system of grazing. Increasing the stocking
rate on the continuously grazed treatment caused a reduction in animal
production per hectare whereas on the rotationally grazed treatment, the
same high stocking rate caused a substantial increase in production per
hectare. This was probably caused by the reduction of 35% in liveweight
gain per animal from increasing the stocking rate on the continuously
grazed treatment, whereas there was a reduction of only 18% on the
rotationally grazed treatment. Carcass weights showed the same trend as
the liveweights with a slightly higher percentage killout for the
rotationally grazed animals (Table 2)

Over the three years there was a similar variation in the
digestibility of the herbage on offer over the season. In 1980
digestibility was considerably lower on the continuously grazed treatment

TABLE 2   Carcass weights and percentage kill out

	Liveweight kg	Carcass weight kg	% killout
Continuous grazing			
LSR	393	204	51.7
HSR	337	177	52.7
Rotational grazing			
LSR	402	217	53.9
HSR	379	203	53.4
Standard deviation	14.59***	17.47*	0.997***

than that on offer on the rotationally grazed plots (Fig.1). On average throughout the year, the continuously grazed treatment offered herbage with a digestibility of 69.3% OMD while the rotationally grazed treatment offered herbage with a digestibility of 76.6% OMD. There was no significant difference however, in the digestibility of the herbage selected by the animals which averaged 79.6% OMD from the continuously grazed pasture and 80.7% OMD from the rotationally grazed system.

Measurements of grazing time showed that, at high stocking rates, the continuously grazed animals grazed for 10.9 hours while those on the rotationally grazed system grazed for only 8 hours (Table 3). Animals were changed to a new paddock at 14.00h and between then and dusk had similar grazing times as those on the continuously grazed system. During the second period of grazing however, the rotationally grazed animals only grazed for half the length of time of those on the set stocked system.

The distance walked by animals on both systems showed the same pattern as the time spent grazing. The continuously grazed animals walked more than 2.7 times as much as the rotationally grazed animals during a full days grazing. The distribution of distance walked between the afternoon and morning grazing periods also followed closely the pattern of grazing during the same periods. There was no significant difference between the two systems in the length of time the animals spent lying but the rotationally grazed animals stood for more than twice the time of the continuously grazed animals.

The energy requirements of these various activities have been calculated using the data of Graham (1964a,b). Although those data were for sheep rather than cattle and consequently may not give absolute values

146

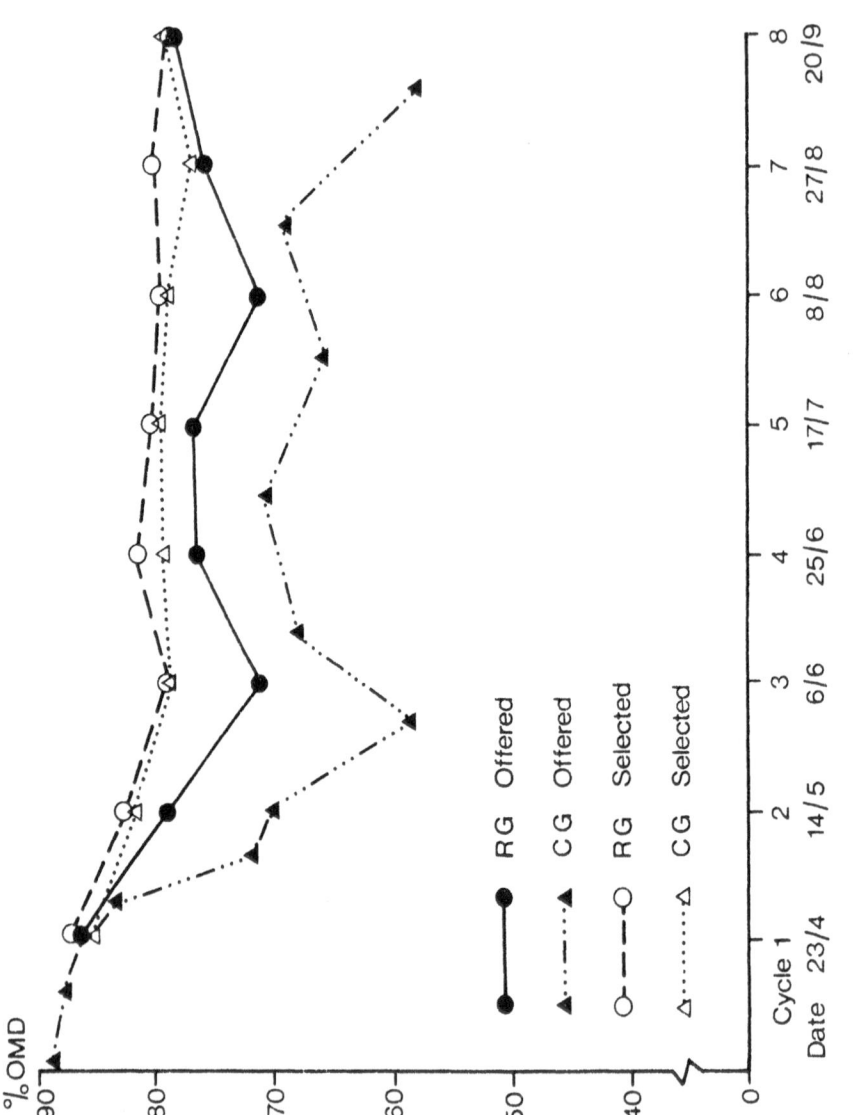

Fig. 1   Digestibility of herbage offered and selected (1980)

TABLE 3   Grazing behaviour and its conversion into energy at high stocking rates

	Grazing min	Walking metres	Standing min	Lying min	Energy (kJ/kg body wt/day)
Continuous grazing	654	5085	94	691	39.4
Rotational grazing	478	1876	197	765	27.3
SE mean and significance	11.9***	156.1***			

of energy expenditure, they allow a comparison to be made between the energy expenditure of the animals on the different treatments.   Table 3 indicates that the continuously grazed animals expended 44% more energy on grazing activity than the rotationally grazed animals.

A summary of the data on digestible organic matter intake and liveweight gain over the three years is shown in Table 4.   At the low stocking rate the continuously grazed animals ate 8% (P<0.001) more than the rotationally grazed animals while at the same time they put on 7% (P<0.001) less weight.   At the high stocking rate although the rotationally grazed animals ate 4% more but they put on 39% (P<0.001) more weight.   The resultant figures for conversion efficiency show that at both stocking rates the continuously grazed animals ate more per unit of liveweight gain than did the rotationally grazed animals, 14% more at the low stocking rate and 25% more at the high stocking rate.

The energy requirements for maintenance and activity were calculated by converting the digestible organic matter intake into total energy intake and subtracting from this the energy requirement for liveweight gain (MAFF,1975).   In all years, and at both stocking rates, the maintenance energy requirement was lower for the animals on the rotationally grazed paddocks than for those on the continuously grazed treatment, by 18% at the low stocking rate and by 11% at the high stocking rate on average over the three years (Table 5).

Correlation analysis showed that over the three years the digestible organic matter intake, DM offered, green material offered and the digestibility of the material offered were all significant factors affecting liveweight gain (Table 6).   The amount of dry matter offered had the least effect of the parameters presented and the digestible organic matter intake the greatest.   However at best, only 66% of the variation in liveweight gain could be explained by changes in intake.   Multiple regression analysis involving the other parameters as well as intake did not significantly increase the correlation.

TABLE 4   Digestible organic matter intake and liveweight gain
(average of 3 years)

	DOMI (g/kg LW/day)	LWG (g/kg LW/day)	DOMI/LWG
Continuous grazing			
LSR	20.94	2.89	7.23
HSR	18.82	1.94	9.70
Rotational grazing			
LSR	19.44	3.11	6.25
HSR	19.52	2.69	7.26
SE mean and significance	0.247***	0.77***	0.381***

TABLE 5   Energy requirements for maintenance and activity

	ME MJ/animal/day			
	1978	1979	1980	Mean
Continuous grazing				
LSR	58.8	50.5	68.6	59.3
HSR	57.5	59.2	67.7	61.5
Rotational grazing				
LSR	45.4	46.2	54.1	48.5
HSR	50.3	51.2	62.1	54.5
SE mean and significance	2.20**	1.74**	2.38**	1.26***

TABLE 6   The influence of intake and the amount and type of material
offered on the liveweight gain of animals (R^2)
(average of 3 years)

	Continuous grazing		Rotational grazing	
	LSR	HSR	LSR	HSR
DOMI	0.637***	0.662***	0.545***	0.565***
DM offered	0.069 NS	0.484***	0.058 NS	0.215*
Green offered	0.466***	0.500***	0.245*	0.268*
% DMD offered	0.560***	0.313*	0.273*	0.281*

LWG expressed as g LWG/kg LW/day; DOMI expressed as g DOM/kg LW/day;
DM offered expressed as g DM/kg LW/day;
Green offered expressed as g green DM/kg LW/day

DISCUSSION

It is now accepted that although different grazing systems can affect the sward by changing factors like tiller density, grazing severity and leaf area, the sward as a whole has considerable compensatory powers of maintaining optimum production. Consequently, Ernst et al (1980) and Hodgson and Wade (1978) have found that this flexibility allows similar levels of dry matter production from a wide range of grazing managements. In this experiment there was no significant difference in the amount of grass produced between the two systems although the high stocking rate always slightly depressed production. This supports the conclusion of Hodgson and Wade (1978) that "annual herbage accumulation is relatively insensitive to variations in grazing management or to variations in stocking rate within the range likely to be of practical interest".

The pattern of liveweight gain was similar to that of previous experiments (Conway, 1963b) which showed an advantage to rotational grazing at high stocking rates. However at high stocking rates, production per animal is depressed while production per unit area is increased, although this might be acceptable in a dairying situation it may not be suitable for the beef producer who has a greater interest in production per animal. Care must be exercised in the interpretation of results and it may be necessary to adopt a level of stocking that will give adequate liveweight gains per hectare while at the same time maintaining animal performance at approximately 1 kg liveweight gain per animal per day.

Much information is available on the energy metabolism of housed farm livestock but less is known about the energy requirements of grazing animals. Estimates range from only slightly above that of housed animals (Corbett et al, 1961; Van Es, 1974) to values for sheep two to three times as great (Coop and Hill, 1962; Lambourne and Reardon, 1963). Van Es calculated that dairy cows have a daily energy requirement which is only 10% higher than stall-fed cows but Graham (1964b) calculated that a 50 kg sheep kept on sparse pasture, 5 km from water, would expend more than eight times as much energy as a sheep on good pasture.

The differences in energy expenditure reported here between the two systems of grazing stress the value of behavioural measurements in explaining differences in comparative grazing trials. The variation in maintenance requirements observed between the different nutritional environments would be enough to severely obscure correlations between food intake and animal performance under normal management.

REFERENCES

Conway, A. 1963a. Effect of grazing management on beef production.
    I. Comparison of three systems of grazing. Ir.J.agric.Res. **2** 87
Conway, A. 1963b. Effect of grazing management on beef production.
    II. Comparison of three stocking rates under three systems of
    grazing.
    Ir. J. agric.Res. **2** 243
Conway, A. 1964. Effect of grazing management on beef production.
    III. Effect of stocking rate and grazing method on carcass
    measurements. Ir. J. agric. Res. **3** 165
Coop, I.E. and Hill, M.K. 1962. The energy requirement of sheep for
    maintenance and gain. J. agric.Sci.,Camb. **58** 187
Corbett, J.L., Langlands, J.P. and Boyne, W.A. 1961. An estimate of the
    energy expended for maintenance by strip grazed dairy cows.
    Proc. 8th Int.Grassld Cong., p.245
Drew, J.P. and Deasy, D. 1937. An investigation into the intensive
    system of grassland management. J. Dept.Agric.,Dublin **24** 3
Ernst,P.,LeDu,Y.L.P. and Carlier,L. 1980. Animal and sward production
    under rotational and continuous grazing management - a critical
    appraisal. Proc. Int. Symp. Eur. Grassld Fed. on the role of nitrogen
    in intensive grassland production, Wageningen, p.119
Es, A.J.M. van 1974. Energy intake and requirement of dairy cows during
    the whole year. Livest. Prod. Sci., **1** 21
Graham, N. McC. 1964a. Energy costs of feeding activities and energy
    expenditure of grazing sheep. Aust. J. agric. Res. **15** 969
Graham, N. McC. 1964b. Maintenance requirements of sheep indoors and at
    pasture. Proc. Aust. Soc. Anim. Prod. **5** 272
Hodgson, J. and Rodriguez, J.M. 1970. The measurement of herbage intake in
    grazing studies. Ann. Rep. GRI, Hurley, p. 132
Hodgson, J. and Wade, M.H. 1978. Grazing systems and herbage
    production.In: Proc. Br. Grassld Soc.,Winter Meeting, p.1.1-1.12
Lambourne, L.J. and Reardon, T.F. 1963. Effect of environment on the
    maintenance requirements of merino wethers. Aust.J. agric.Res. **14** 272
MAFF 1975. Energy allowances and feeding systems for ruminants.
    Technical Bulletin 33, London: Her Majesty's Stationery
    Office,1976,p.5
Marsh, R. 1975. Systems of grazing management for beef cattle. In: Pasture
    utilisation by the grazing animal. Ed. J. Hodgson and D.K.Jackson.
    Occasional Symposium No.8,British Grassland Society,p.119
McCarthy, D. 1979. Milk production from grassland. In:Proc.Milk Production
    Seminar, Moorepark, Ireland
McMeekan, C.P. 1956. Grazing management and animal production. Proc.7th
    Int.Grassld Cong.,p.146
McMeekan, C.P. and Walshe, M.J. 1963. The inter-relationships of grazing
    method and stocking rate in the efficiency of pasture utilisation by
    dairy cattle. J. agric.Sci., Camb. **61** 147
Tilley, J.M.A. and Terry,R.A. 1963. A two-stage technique for the in vitro
    digestion of forage crops. J. Br. Grassld Soc. **18** 108
Williams, C.H.,David,D.J. and Ilsmaa,O. 1962. The determination of chromic
    oxide in faeces samples by atomic absorption spectrophotometry.
    J.agric. Sci.,Camb. **59** 381

CONCENTRATE SUPPLEMENTATION OF GRAZING CATTLE

J.A.C. Meijs

Institute for Livestock Feeding and Nutrition Research (IVVO),

8200 AD Lelystad, The Netherlands

ABSTRACT

A trial was carried out at Lelystad to investigate supplementation effects on herbage intake by grazing dairy cows at variable levels of daily herbage allowance.

Two experiments are described in which twenty-four spring-calving Dutch Friesian cows were allocated to six grazing treatments (two levels of daily herbage allowance x three levels of daily concentrate intake) in a 2 by 3 factorial design. The pre-cut swards consisted predominantly of perennial ryegrass. A two-machine sward-cutting technique was used for estimating herbage intake by cows grazing swards for 3 or 4 days with correction for herbage accumulation during grazing. Experiment 1 was carried out during 16 weeks of the grazing season of 1981; experiment 2 during 18 weeks of 1982.

Daily herbage OM allowances in both experiments were 16 and 25 kg per cow above 4 cm cutting height. Daily concentrate OM intake ranged from 0.8 to 5.6 kg per cow. The effect of concentrates on herbage intake differed significantly between allowances. At the low allowance level and at daily OM concentrate intakes of 0.8, 3.2 and 5.6 kg per cow, daily herbage OM intake was 10.9, 10.6 and 10.4 kg per cow respectively and mean substitution rate of herbage by concentrates was only 0.1. At the high allowance level and at daily OM concentrate intakes of 0.8, 3.2 and 5.6 kg per cow daily herbage OM intake was 14.8, 13.6 and 12.4 kg per cow respectively and mean substitution rate was 0.5 kg OM herbage/kg OM concentrates.

INTRODUCTION

The effect of supplements on the level of production by grazing cattle may depend on: the quantity and quality of herbage consumed when it is offered as the sole feed, the nutrient requirements of the animal and the quantity and quality of supplementary nutrient fed.

Most of the supplementation trials in the literature report only data on quantity of supplement fed and on animal production. Quantity of herbage offered has seldom been determined in animal production trials, but it can be expected that herbage allowance has been high (Leaver et al., 1968)

Stocking rate has increased during the last decade in the Netherlands. There is not yet sufficient evidence from experiments with grazing cattle to be able to judge the responses that can be expected from feeding of concentrates when herbage is scarce. Therefore trials to determine the effects of concentrate supplementation at variable levels of daily herbage allowance were carried out at Lelystad.

In the trials reported here quantities of herbage offered and quantities of concentrates consumed were varied. The quality of herbage and concentrates was measured. It was aimed to supply highly digestible herbage of constant quality, together with a low-protein concentrate compound containing nearly 100% of by-products of the feed industry.

Dutch grassland is mainly used by dairy cattle, and dairy cows were used in the grazing experiments. But because the principal effects of herbage allowance on substitution rate are probably the same for different types of cattle our work on cows is also likely to apply to beef cattle.

Highly productive spring-calving cows with high nutrient requirements were used, compared with many experiments in the literature, in which low yielding cows have been used and a low response to supplementation recorded (Leaver et al, 1968)

MATERIALS AND METHODS

Experimental design

Three levels of concentrates and two levels of daily herbage allowance were compared in a 2 by 3 factorial design. The daily herbage allowances were 16 (L) and 24 (H) kg organic matter (OM) per cow above a stubble height of 4 cm. The concentrates were fed in the milking parlour in equal amounts at the two milking times at rates of 1, 3 and 5 kg per day in 1981 (Experiment 1) and 1, 4 and 7 kg per day in 1982 (Experiment 2). Four groups of cows were available. As is shown for the first six weeks of Experiment 2 (Table 1) the groups changed to another treatment every week. In Experiment 1, a comparable design was used combining two low herbage allowance and two high herbage allowance levels each week; but with concentrate intakes of 1, 3 and 5 kg per cow per day. Each week consisted of a 4 day preliminary period where the treatments were applied, followed by a 3 day experimental grazing period during which the mean intake of groups of dairy cows was determined. The first trial started 14 May 1981 and lasted for 16 weeks, the second trial started 27 May 1982 and lasted for 18 weeks.

Animals

Twenty-four Dutch Friesian cows were used in both experiments. No heifers were used. The annual milk production of the cows in the previous lactation was 6400 kg (Experiment 1) and 6500 kg (Experiment 2). The 24

TABLE 1   Design for the first six weeks of experiment 2

| Animal group | Experimental period (week) | | | | | |
	1	2	3	4	5	6
I	L4[1])	H7	L1	H4	L7	H1
II	L7	H1	L4	H7	L1	H4
III	H1	L4	H7	L1	H4	L7
IV	H4	L7	H1	L4	H7	L1

1) L and H : low (16) and high (24) daily herbage OM allowance
   (>4 cm)
1, 4 and 7 : concentrates offered per cow (kg/day)

cows were classified in blocks of comparable age, calving date, milk production in the previous lactation and milk production during the first weeks of the current lactation, and were then allotted at random to 4 grazing groups of six animals. In 1981 the average calving date was 29 March, average weight was 579 kg and they produced on average 25.5 kg of 4% fat-corrected milk per day during the trial; in 1982 the corresponding figures were 27 March, 575 kg and 22.2 kg FCM per day respectively.

Feed

The concentrates included dried beet pulp (250 g/kg), tapioca (230 g/kg), maize (120 g/kg), linseed expeller (150 g/kg), coconut expeller (120 g/kg), cane molasses (100 g/kg) and minerals/vitamins (30 g/kg).

The main component of the sward on all pastures was perennial ryegrass (700-900 g/kg). Each grazing plot was used experimentally for only one week during the season; in the rest of the season it was used by the farm herd. In Experiment 1 and in the first 15 weeks of Experiment 2 each plot was cut at the defoliation prior to the experimental grazing. In the last 3 weeks of Experiment 2 each plot was grazed at the previous defoliation and the residual herbage was topped and removed. The plots received about 80 kg Nitrogen per ha, immediately after the previous harvest. During the first eight weeks of both experiments the swards were top-dressed with 15-20 kg MgO per ha, at the start of each grazing period.

Measurements

The cows in both groups grazed grass swards of the same herbage mass per unit area but contrasting daily herbage allowances were achieved by using grazed areas, one 50% larger than the other for the same grazing period and number of cows. Allowances were based on estimates of herbage mass made by cutting 10 strips with a motor scythe on each grazed pasture just before the start of grazing, and correcting for herbage accumulation during grazing (see below)

A two-step cutting technique was used to estimate daily herbage intake (Meijs, 1981; Meijs et al, 1982). Ten strips of herbage were cut with a motor scythe followed by a lawnmower (cutting height 3 cm) at the start (strip length 12 m) and finish (strip length 15 m) of the grazing period. Herbage intake was corrected for realized herbage accumulation during grazing. The realized herbage accumulation was measured by cutting 10 strips from a fenced ungrazed area at the start and finish of the grazing period and applying Linehan's equation (see Meijs et al, 1982) for calculating the factor between herbage accumulation on the fenced ungrazed area and on the grazed area. The ten samples of the herbage cut with both machines at the start and finish of grazing were dried separately after subsampling and bulked for chemical analyses and in-vitro OM digestibility determination (Meijs, 1981).

RESULTS

The mean chemical composition and net energy content, based on in vitro OM digestibility estimates of the concentrates fed and of the herbage offered, are given in Table 2. The mean protein content of the concentrates fed was somewhat higher in 1981 than in 1982 due to a mistake in the mixing of the concentrate components in the factory in one of the five batches in 1981. As in the practical farm situation in the Netherlands the supplement was relatively low in protein, high in energy and high in starch and sugars. The chemical composition and nutritive value of the herbage offered above 4 cm in both experiments were very similar; the protein content and the OM digestibility were high.

In total 64 and 72 intake observations were obtained in experiments 1 and 2 respectively. Due to sick cows, 2 and 3 intake measurements were excluded from tables and analyses in experiments 1 and 2. Difficulties in cutting conditions (adhesion of herbage to the lawnmower) during pre- and post-grazing sampling leading to systematic errors in estimates of intake (Meijs, 1981), occurred during 9 and 5 measurements respectively; these data were also excluded. So 53 (Experiment 1) and 64 (Experiment 2) reliable intake estimates remained (in total n = 117).

TABLE 2   Chemical composition and net energy content of concentrates fed and of herbage offered above 4 cm in g/kg organic matter.

	Concentrates 1981	1982	Herbage 1981	1982
Crude protein (cp)	172	152	268	270
Crude fibre (cf)	103	113	240	252
Crude fat (cfat)	42	31	-	-
Sugars	104	117	126	106
Starch	254	297	-	-
Neutral detergent residue (NDR)	297	277	531	561
Digestible crude protein (dcp)	130	111	215	217
Digestible organic matter (doM)	835	858	782	772
Net energy (VEM/kg)	1161	1176	1068	1055

The mean figures of the realised treatments are given in Table 3. Nearly all the concentrates fed were consumed as intended. There was good agreement too between the intended levels of daily herbage allowance (16 and 24 kg OM/cow above 4 cm) and the realised treatments (Table 3). The mean daily herbage intake per treatment is included in Table 3. There was a strong positive effect of herbage allowance on daily herbage intake. The effect of concentrates on herbage intake depended on the allowance level. The mean data of Table 3 are not corrected for week and animal group effects. Because of excluded data the distribution of treatments over weeks and groups was not balanced. Moreover daily herbage allowance varied somewhat between weeks, due to differences between the expected and the actual herbage accumulation during the grazing period. Therefore herbage intake was analysed by multiple regression using the variables year, period, group, herbage allowance, concentrate consumption and several combinations of linear, curvilinear and interaction terms. Statistical analyses of the experiments separately are presented in the extensive reports of the trials (Meijs, 1982, 1983a). Here only the results of the analysis of the combined data are given. The best fitting model for the total data, after correction for year, period and animal group effects is given graphically in Figure 1, at daily herbage allowances ranging from 15 to 26 kg OM/day and at daily intakes of concentrates of 1, 4 and 7 kg (corresponding with 0.8, 3.2 and 6.4 kg OM). Analysis of regression showed

TABLE 3   Effect of daily herbage allowance and concentrate intake
           on herbage OM intake (all expressed kg/cow/day);n = 117

	Daily herbage allowance (kg OM per cow >4 cm)	
	16.4	24.9
Experiment 1 Intake of concentrates		
0.8	11.1	14.6
2.4	11.0	14.0
3.8	11.4	12.5
	16.1	24.7
Experiment 2 Intake of concentrates		
0.8	11.6	15.1
3.2	11.8	13.2
5.6	10.6	12.0

significant effects of herbage allowance ($P<0.025$) and of concentrate intake ($P<0.025$) on herbage intake. The negative effect of concentrates on herbage intake increased at higher levels of daily herbage allowance and a significant ($P<0.01$) allowance:concentrate interaction was shown. Predictions of mean herbage intakes at four allowance levels using the best regression model are made in Table 4.   Mean substitution or replacement rate, defined as the decrease of herbage OM intake per kg OM of concentrates, is also given in Table 4.   Substitution rate from 0.8 to 3.2 kg OM of concentrates did not differ significantly from substitution rate from 3.2 to 5.6 kg OM of concentrates.   The substitution rate increased significantly ($P<0.01$) with daily herbage allowances.

The digestibility and net energy content of herbage ingested (for method of calculation see Meijs, 1981, p.157) were 4–5% higher than those of herbage offered above 4 cm, showing that animals consumed minimum herbage in the layer of 4–7 cm; this was also evident from measurements of sward height at the end of grazing.   There was no significant effect of treatment on in vitro digestibility or nutritive value of herbage ingested so that relative differences in intake of nutrients from herbage between treatments were comparable to those for intake of organic matter from herbage.

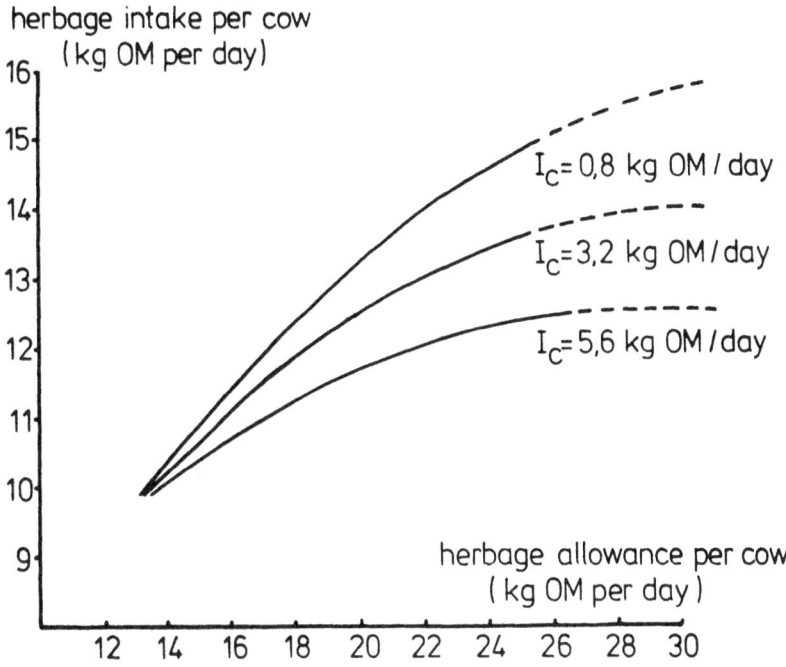

Fig. 1   The effect of herbage allowance upon daily herbage intake
at different levels of daily intake of concentrates (I_C)

TABLE 4   Predicted herbage OM intakes and substitution rates from
the regression model

| | Daily herbage OM allowance (kg/cow > 4 cm) | | | |
	15	20	25	30
Daily concentrate intake (kg OM)	Daily herbage intake (kg OM)			
0.8	10.9	13.2	14.8	15.7
3.2	10.6	12.5	13.6	14.0
5.6	10.4	11.7	12.4	12.4
Mean substitution rate from 0.8 to 5.6 kg OM of concentrates	0.11 (0.07)*	0.30 (0.05)	0.50 (0.07)	0.69 (0.10)

* The figure in brackets is the standard deviation of the mean substitution rate.

The in vitro OM digestibility of concentrates and herbage ingested were about equal. At an increase of concentrate consumption of 6 kg (c.4.1 kg DOM) the intake of DOM from the total ration increased by 3.4 kg (=34%) at the low allowance and by 1.6 kg (=12%) at the high allowance respectively.

DISCUSSION

The two-step sward cutting technique used to estimate herbage intake in these experiments has been discussed extensively by Meijs (1981) and Meijs et al (1982). On pre-cut pastures it was possible to estimate mean herbage intake with a coefficient of variation of 5%. An advantage of the method is that the measurements also provide information on the herbage mass and allowance. The major disadvantages of the technique are that it is limited to mean intake estimates for groups of cows and to rotational grazing methods Moreover it requires a high input of labour, especially on less homogenous swards, e.g. on repeatedly grazed swards. An advantage of the sward method is that supplementation of grazing animals does not affect the herbage intake measurement technique in contrast to the methods based on digestibility estimates (Milne et al, 1980)

In most conditions the feeding of supplements does result in some increase in milk yield and therefore the observed intake of grass is confounded with differences in output. This can be partially alleviated experimentally by the use of of short-term trials like the change-over design adopted here. In previous experiments (Meijs, 1981) residual effects after treatment periods varying from one to three weeks could not be shown and the effects of herbage allowance on intake could be established with treatment periods of one week.

The strong positive effect of daily herbage allowance on daily herbage intake has been shown before (Meijs,1981; 1983b). Compared with the literature the allowance effects on herbage intake at Lelystad were large, which might be attributed to the use of highly productive cows, to the application of grazing periods of 3-4 days and to the measurement of herbage allowance above a cutting height of 4 cm (Meijs, 1981). From behavioural studies it has been shown that the major factor diminishing intake at a low allowance level was the size of bites ingested (Meijs,1981)

These experiments have shown that the effect of concentrates on herbage intake of the grazing cows depends on the level of daily herbage allowance. No reports of trials with grazing dairy cows in which both herbage allowance and concentrate supply were varied have been found.Recently Hijink et al (1982) in several zero-grazing experiments with dairy cows showed that when herbage intake was low, concentrate supplementation hardly affected herbage intake; but when the intake of herbage offered as the sole feed was high, the substitution of herbage by concentrates was also high. A comparison of substitution rates in the

zero-grazing trials of Hijink et al (1982) and in the grazing trials
reported here is made in Table 5. Because of the expression of zero grazing
results in dry matter the OM intake data at pasture were transformed into
DM by multiplying by 1.11. Level of concentrate consumption significantly
affected substitution rate indoors but in the grazing trials this could not

TABLE 5   Prediction of mean substitution rates indoors
(Hijink et al, 1982) or at pasture (Experiments 1 and 2);
all data expressed in dry matter

		Daily herbage DM allowance at pasture (kg/cow, > 4 cm)		
		16.6	22.2	27.7
Herbage intake (DM)	stall	12.1	14.9	16.9
when no concentrates	pasture	12.1	14.9	16.9
are consumed				
Mean substitution rate	stall	0.22	0.41	0.54
from 0 to 3.6 kg DM of	pasture	0.11	0.30	0.50
concentrates				
Mean substitution rate	stall	0.35	0.54	0.67
from 0 to 6.3 kg DM of	pasture	0.11	0.30	0.50
concentrates				

be shown with up to 7 kg concentrate per day. At a concentrate range from
0 to 3.6 kg DM the mean substitution rate indoors was 0.04 to 0.11 higher
than at pasture and not significant. At a concentrate range from 0 to 6.3
kg DM the difference in substitution rate between stall and pasture
increased to significant levels, varying from 0.17 to 0.24. The difference
in substitution rates between stall-fed and grazing cows might be explained
by differences in intake during the 3-day grazing intake period since,
especially at low levels of daily herbage allowance, herbage intake
declines rapidly during a grazing period while there is no systematic trend
in herbage intake between days indoors.

The effects of the factors influencing substitution rate in- and out
doors may partly be related to the difference between the intake of
nutrients from herbage and the animal's requirement especially for net
energy. When herbage allowance does not meet the animal's requirements the
substitution of herbage is low (eg at a low herbage allowance);when the
allowance exceeds requirements substitution of herbage is high. In these
trials the intake of nutrients from herbage was varied. Information on the
effects of variations in nutrient requirement due to variations in milk or

meat production on substitution rate is scarce and more experiments are necessary.

The concentrates used contained a high level of the readily fermentable carbohydrates, starch and sugars. A high intake of such concentrates over a long period might lead to a disturbed rumen fermentation, rumen acidosis and low milk fat syndrome, especially when herbage intake is restricted. More research on herbage intake and rumen fermentation in the long term on grazing cows supplemented with concentrates of different chemical compositions is in progress at the Institute.

REFERENCES

Hijink, J.W.F., Le Du, Y.L.P., Meijs, J.A.C. and Meijer, A.B. 1982
    Supplementation of the grazing dairy cow. Report 141.
    Institute for Livestock Feeding and Nutrition Research, Lelystad,
    The Netherlands.
Leaver, J.D., Campling,R.C. and Holmes,W. 1968. Use of supplementary feeds
    for grazing dairy cows. Dairy Science Abstracts, **30** 355-361.
Meijs, J.A.C. 1981. Herbage intake by grazing dairy cows.
    Agricultural Research Reports 909, Wageningen:Pudoc.
Meijs, J.A.C. 1982. The influence of concentrate supplementation on
    herbage intake by grazing dairy cows. 1. Report of the experiment on
    herbage intake in 1981. Report 143 Institute for Livestock
    Feeding and Nutrition Research, Lelystad, The Netherlands.
Meijs, J.A.C. 1983a. The influence of concentrate supplementation on
    herbage intake by grazing dairy cows. 2. Report of the experiment on
    herbage intake in 1982. Report 149 Institute for Livestock Feeding
    and Nutrition Research, Lelystad, The Netherlands.
Meijs, J.A.C. 1983b. The effect of herbage mass and allowance upon the
    herbage intake by grazing dairy cows. Proceedings XIVth
    International Grassland Congress, Kentucky, 1981, pp.667-670.
Meijs, J.A.C., Walters, R.J.K. and Keen,A. 1982. Sward methods. In:
    Leaver, J.D. (ed.) Herbage Intake Handbook.pp.11-36, British Grassland
    Society, Hurley, England.
Milne, J.A., Maxwell,T.J. and Souter, W. 1980. Effect of supplementary
    feeding and herbage mass on the intake and performance of grazing
    ewes in early lactation. Anim. Prod. **32** 185-195.

A TECHNIQUE FOR THE MEASUREMENT OF GRAZING BEHAVIOUR

P.D. Penning and D.F. Osbourn

The Grassland Research Institute, Hurley, Maidenhead, Berks, SL6 5LR

ABSTRACT
   Equipment to sense and record the jaw movements of grazing sheep is described. The recorded analogue signals are converted to digital form and analysed in a Midas 3 microprocessor. The microprocessor analysis differentiates between jaw movements devoted to prehension and mastication during eating, ruminating and idling, and summates both the jaw movements and time devoted to each action. Preliminary observations suggest that the ratio of time devoted to prehension and mastication is far more sensitive to variation in herbage availability than is the total time spent eating.

   The grazing behaviour of herbivorous animals is measured to obtain an understanding of the animal's reaction to a sward, the ease or difficulty with which the animal prehends its food and the effect this has upon selection within the sward, voluntary food intake and energy expenditure. Such observations may be of value also in understanding the response of the sward to grazing and hence lead to the improvement of management practices.

   The equipment developed at the Grassland Research Institute to measure grazing behaviour and to validate its accuracy has been described in detail by Penning (1983). The transducer sensing the movements of the jaw comprises a silicon rubber tube expanded in chloroform and allowed to shrink on to a uniformly packed filling of carbon granules with turret tag electrodes inserted at each end. When a voltage is applied across the cylinder of carbon granules the resistance, and hence the voltage, changes linearly with the extension of the cylinder.

   This transducer is fabricated into a circle which forms the nose-band of a simple head collar and senses any movement of the lower jaw as an extension of the transducer. The leads from the transducer are connected via a pulse width modulation amplifier to a miniature tape recorder mounted on a saddle retained on the animal's back by a simple harness. The circuits of the amplifier provide automatic control of base line drift and accommodate any small differences in the sensitivity of the transducers, and the recorder operates for 24 hours using a C120 cassette.

   The cassettes are played back through a PB2 playback unit and a PM3 amplifier at 60 times the recording speed. The replayed signals can be displayed on an oscillograph or permanently recorded using an ultra-violet oscillograph (Fig. 1). In order to automatically analyse the signals the cassette is replayed via an analogue digital convertor into a Midas 3 microprocessor which is programmed using 8080 Assembly language to differentiate between jaw movements devoted to prehension, mastication and rumination, to count jaw movements, and to summate the time spent on each action. The decoded information is then printed out in the form shown in Fig.2 which presents the type of action at one minute intervals and then summates for 24 hours the number of jaw movements and time devoted to each action.

This equipment has proved extremely robust and reliable in use in the field. It provides an accurate, completely automated estimate of the time spent eating, ruminating and idling and, in addition, the time devoted to prehension and to mastication during eating. The equipment is simple to attach to a variety of sheep, and to operate, and has been shown to be more accurate than measurements obtained by mercury switches (O'Shea, 1969) or accelerometers (Chambers et al.1981)

Further work is in progress to develop an algorithm to analyse the jaw movements of cattle, and to investigate the relationship between the ratio of prehension to mastication jaw-movements and bite size (Stobbs, 1973) and, together with total time spent grazing, the feasibility of predicting voluntary food intake (Chacon, Stobbs and Sandland,1976)

The same recording equipment has been used to estimate heart rate, while transducers could also be developed to estimate some leg movements and hence distance walked and other physical and behavioural responses by the animal to stress.

The Grassland Research Institute is financed through the Agricultural Research Council. The work forms part of a commission from the Ministry of Agriculture, Fisheries and Food.

REFERENCES

Chacon,E., Stobbs, T.H. and Sandland, R.L. 1976. Estimation of herbage consumption by grazing cattle using measurements of eating behaviour. Journal of the British Grassland Society **31** 81-87

Chambers, A.R.M., Hodgson,J. and Milne, J.A. 1981. The development of equipment for the automatic recording of ingestive behaviour in sheep and cattle. Grass and Forage Science **36** 97-105

O'Shea, J. 1969. Evaluation of a simple device for measuring the time animals spend grazing. Irish Journal of Agric. Res. **8** 329-333

Penning, P.D. 1983. A technique to record automatically some aspects of grazing and ruminating behaviour in sheep. Grass and Forage Science, **38** 86-96

Stobbs, T.H. 1973. The effect of plant structure on intake of tropical pastures. I. Variation in the bite size of grazing cattle. Australian Journal of Agricultural Research **24** 821-829

163

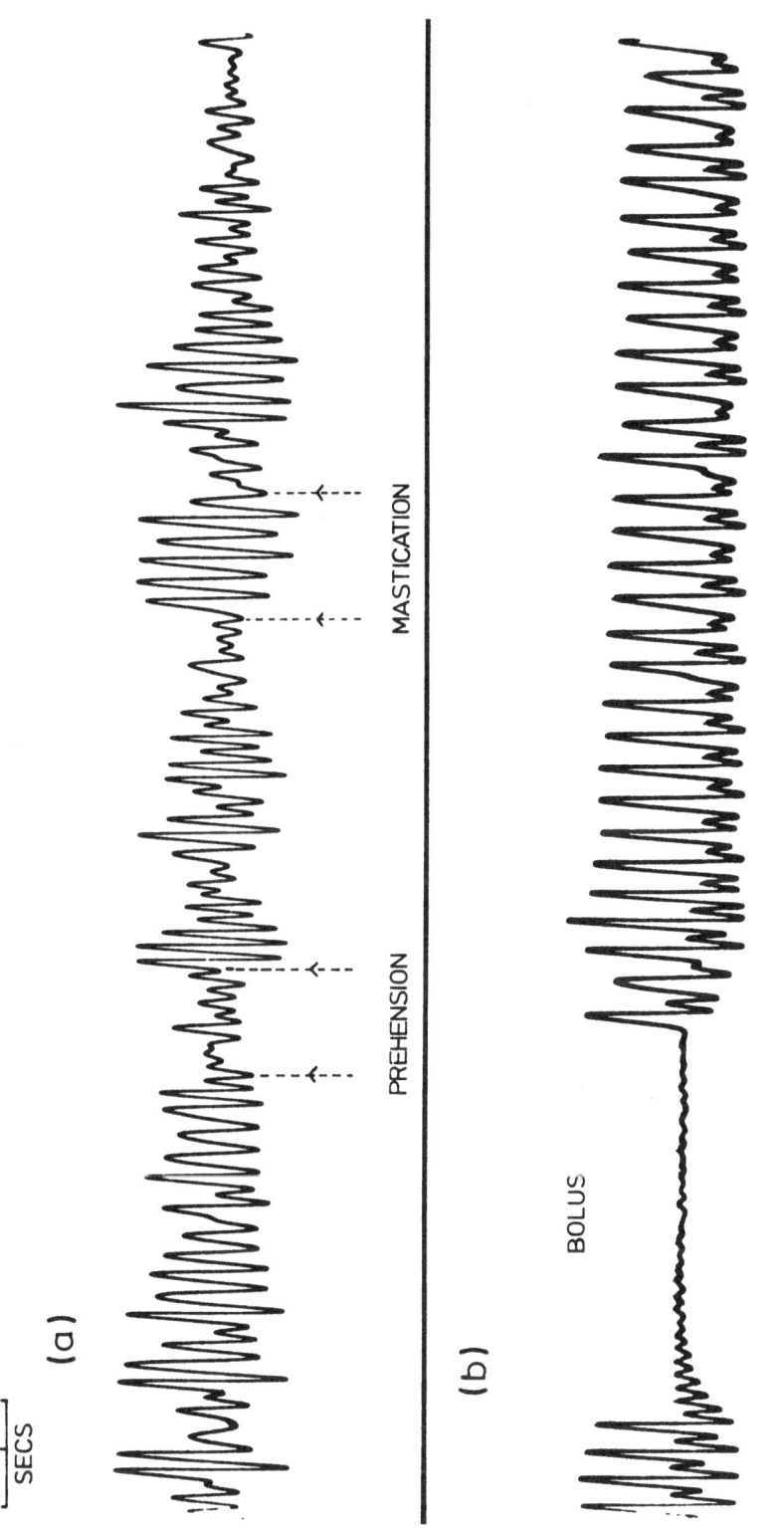

Fig. 1   Oscillograph traces of the jaw movements of a sheep (a) grazing (b) ruminating

EWE 8 11-12/7/82 START 09.49 TURN OUT 09.59 FINISH 09.33   PLOT 40

```
09.00                                                  IIIIEIRRREE
10.00    EEEEEEEEEEEIIEEEEEEEIEEEEEEEEEEEEEEEEEEEEEEEEEEEEEEEEEEEEEEE
11.00    EEEEEEEEEEEEEEEEEEEEEEEEEEEEEEEEEEEEEEEEEEEEEEEEEEEEEEEEEEEEE
12.00    EEEEEEEEEEEEEEEEEEEEEEEEEEEEEEEEEEEEEEEEEEEEEEEEEEEEEEEEEEEEE
13.00    EEEERRRRRRRRREEERRRRRRRRRRRRRRRRRRRRRRRRRRRRRIREEEEEEEEEEEEEEE
14.00    EEEEEEEEEEEEEEEEEEEEEEEEEEEEEEEEEEEEEEEEEEEEEEEEIIIIRRRIRIRI
15.00    IIIRRRIRRRIEEEEEEEEEEEEEEEEEEEEEEEEEEEEEEEEEEEEEEEEEEEEEEEEE
16.00    EEEEEEEEEEEEEEEEEIEEEEEEEEEEEEEEEEEEEEEEEEEEEEEEEEEEEEEEEEEE
17.00    EEEEEEEEEEEEEEEEEEEEEEEEEEEEEEEIIIIIIIIEEEEEEEEEEEEEEEEEEEE
18.00    EEEEEEEEEEEEEEEEEEEEEEEEEEEEEEEEEEEEEEEEEEEEEEEEEEEEEEEEEEEI
19.00    RRIIIIIRRRRRRRRRRRRRRRRRRRRRIIIIIIIIEEEEEEEEEEEEEEEEEEEEEEE
20.00    EEEEEEEEEEEEEEEEEEEEEEEEEEEEEEEEEEEEEEEEEEEEEEEEEEEEEEEEEEEEE
21.00    EEEEEEEEEEEEEEEEEEEEEEEEEEEEEEEEEEEEEEEEEEEEEERIRRRRRRIRIIRRR
22.00    RRRRRIIIIIIIIIIIIIIIIIIIIIIIIIIIIIEIIIIIIIIIIIIIIIIIIIIIIIIII
23.00    IIIIIIIIIIIIIIIRRRRRRRRRRRRRRRIRRRRRRRRRIIIIIIIIIIIIIIIIIIIIII
24.00    IIIIIIIIIIIIIIIIIIIIIIIIIRRRRRRRRRRRRRRRIIRIRRRRRRRRRRRIIIIR
01.00    RRRRRIIIIIIIIIIIIIIIIIIIIIIIIRRRRRRRRRRRRRRRRRRRRRRRRRRRRRRRR
02.00    RRIRRRRRRRRRRRRRRRRRRRRRRRRRRRRIIIIIIIEEEEEEEEEEEEEEEEEEEEEE
03.00    EIRRRRRRRRRRRRRRRRRRRRRRRRRRRRRRRRRRRRRRRRRRRRRRRRRRRRRRRRRR
04.00    RRRRRRRRRRRRRRRRRRIIIIIIIIIRRRRRRRRRRERRRRRRRRRRRRRRRRRRRRRRR
05.00    RRRRRRRRRRIIEEEEEEEEEEEEEEEEEEEEEEEEEEEEEEEEEIRRRRRRRRRRRRRR
06.00    RRRRRRRRRRRRRRRRRRRRRRIIIIIIIIIIIRRRRRRRRRRRRRRRRRRRRRRRRRRRR
07.00    IRRRRRRRRRRRRRRREEEEEEEEEEEEEEEEEEEEEEEEEEEEEEEEEEEEEEEEEEEE
08.00    EEEEEEEEEEEEEEEEEEEEEEEEEEEEEEEEEEEEEEEEEEEERRRRRRRRRRRRRRRRR
09.00    RRRRRRRRRRRRRRRRRRRRRRRREIEEIIIIIIII
```

1424 MINUTES OF DATA RECORDED

751 MINUTES EATING   52.7% OF THE DAY
58850 PREHENSION BITES   MEAN 78 PER MINUTE
53287 MASTICATION BITES,   MEAN 71 PER MINUTE

TOTAL 112137 JAW MOVEMENTS MEAN 149 PER MINUTE

23494 EATING UNITS   MEAN 31 PER MINUTE
MEAN OF 2.5 PREHENSION BITES AND 2.3 MASTICATION BITES PER EATING UNIT
MEAN OF 0.91 MASTICATION BITES PER PREHENSION BITE

435 MINUTES RUMINATING   30.5% OF THE DAY
35137 CHEWS   MEAN 81 PER MINUTE

640 PAUSES BETWEEN BOLUS   MEAN LENGTH 8.9 SECONDS
MEAN FREQUENCY 1.5 PER RUMINATING MINUTE
MEAN OF 54 CHEWS PER BOLUS
ACTUAL RUMINATING RATE   106 CHEWS PER MINUTE

238 MINUTES IDLING   16.7% OF THE DAY
3410 JAW MOVEMENTS   MEAN 14 PER MINUTE

A GRAND TOTAL OF 150684 JAW MOVEMENTS IN THE DAY.

Fig.2 24 h record of jaw movements of a sheep as decoded and summated
by the microprocessor E = eating; R = ruminating; I = idling

THE EFFECT OF STOCKING RATE AND SIZE OF ANIMAL ON HERBAGE INTAKE AND ANIMAL PERFORMANCE

J.L.F. Zoby and W. Holmes

Wye College, University of London, Ashford, Kent, UK

Large, medium and small cattle (2 of each) grazed together in 4 replications of plots at two stocking rates (48 cattle in all). Feed intake was measured by faecal index methods and contemporary grazing observations were made. In the spring stocking rates were 6 and 12 cattle per ha and the following data were recorded:

SPRING GRAZING

Low stocking rate   Herbage mass 4470 kg/ha, 746 kg/animal

Animal	Lwt kg	Daily gain kg	Herbage OMI kg/d	Bite size mg/kg $W^{0.75}$
Large	624	1.6	10.7	3.1
Medium	432	1.9	8.8	3.0
Small	163	1.4	5.8	3.1
SE mean	28	0.16	0.36	0.14

High stocking rate   Herbage mass 2140 kg/ha, 178 kg/animal

Animal	Lwt kg	Daily gain kg	Herbage OMI kg/d	Bite size mg/kg $W^{0.75}$
Large	639	0.7	6.4	1.6
Medium	447	1.1	7.5	1.8
Small	165	1.2	5.2	2.2
SE Mean	28	0.16	0.36	0.14

Intake of digestible organic matter (DOMI) was related to animal factors as follows:

Average OMI kg/d = $0.63 + 0.023\ W^{0.75} + 1.583$ LWG

$R^2 = 0.75$ RSD = 0.88   n = 23

In summer the stocking rates were 3.6 and 7.2 cattle per ha. The grazing observations for both seasons are shown in the figure.

166

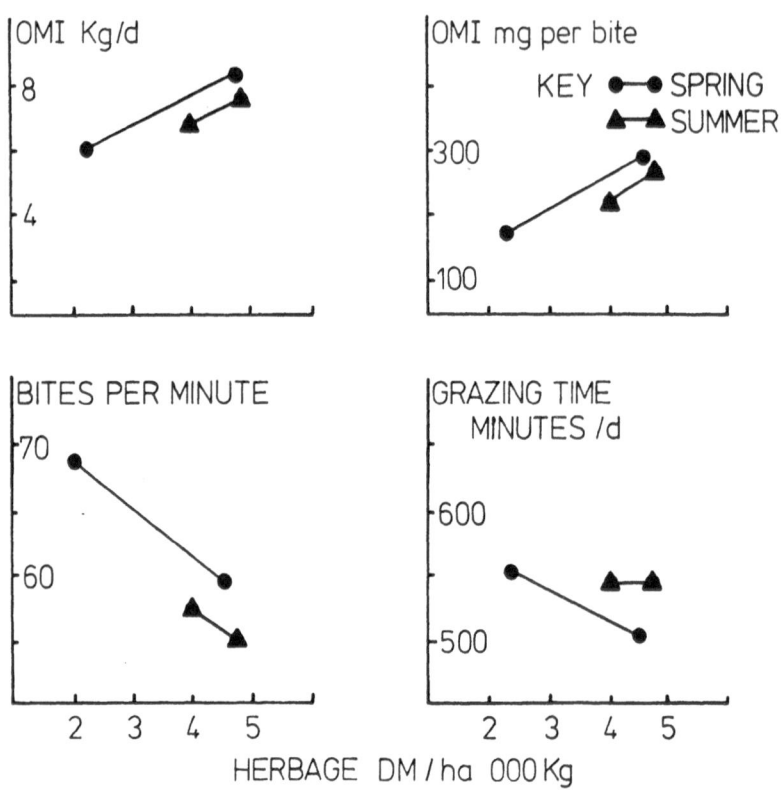

Grazing observations (averages for 24 cattle)

Herbage mass had a profound effect on herbage intake, and all the grazing observations varied accordingly. Similar responses have been shown for sheep by Hodgson (1981)

REFERENCES
Hodgson, J. (1981) p.34 In: Biennial Report 1979-1981, The Hill Farming Research Organisation, Edinburgh
Zoby, J.L.F. PhD thesis, University of London. Factors affecting herbage intake and grazing behaviour in cattle.
Zoby, J.L.F.and Holmes, W. 1983. The influence of size of animal and stocking rate on the herbage intake and grazing behaviour of cattle. J. agric.Sci. 100 139-148

HEIFER PERFORMANCE ON HIGH PASTURES AND DIGESTIBILITY OF PASTURE GRASS

M. Pinosa, E. Tibaldi and U. Fazzini
Istituto di Produzione Animale, Università degli Studi, 33100 Udine, Italy

INTRODUCTION

In Italy about two thirds of the areas devoted to agriculture and forestry are located in mountain and hill zones (ISTAT, 1982). In the last thirty years these areas have been slowly abandoned. Among the possibilities to restore these areas to agriculture, the re-introduction of suckler herds of beef cattle could be of interest. This production system could be advantageous because of the availability of low cost grazing land but most Italian farmers lack knowledge of pastures and herd management. The present research has been to study some problems of pasture utilization in hill areas with beef cattle. In particular the chemical composition and nutritive value of a native pasture located on the Prealpine hills in the NE of Italy has been examined. At the same time the effects of rotation vs continuous grazing and of previous experience of heifers to grazing have been studied.

MATERIALS AND METHODS

The trials were performed in Spring-Summer 1981, on a farm situated at 700 m above sea-level.

The chemical composition and productivity of the pasture were estimated by representative samples drawn from grazing paddocks (15 sampling areas/ha).

Two in vivo digestibility trials (complete balance ingesta-excreta) were carried out, using four Simmental bulls of about 300 kg liveweight, whose daily ration, at maintenance level, was exclusively constituted of pasture grass cut from the rotational paddocks. Chemical analyses were performed on oven dried feedstuffs and faeces following the methodology suggested by A.O.A.C. (1970); structural carbohydrates were evaluated according to Goering and Van Soest (1970).

A grazing trial was conducted with 20 Angus cross heifers (LW 322 kg) born in November-December 1980, half of which were previously accustomed to pasture. On 20 May 1981 two groups of ten heifers, balanced for their previous experience in grazing, were assigned to either rotational or continuous grazing. Due to a fall in forage yield following drought during the second half of July, the rotationally grazed paddocks were opened on 5 August. Liveweights of the heifers were recorded after 12 hours fasting at intervals through the season.

RESULTS AND DISCUSSION

On the basis of grass sampling in Spring 1981, the pasture contained Graminaceae (53-72%) cover, Leguminosae (13-21%) and Compositae (8-16%). The proportion of undesirable plants (Cardus sp., Cirsum sp., Sambucus ebulus, Pteridium aquilium) was normal for a semi-abandoned pasture.

Productivity was 3.2 and 1.9 t of DM/ha respectively for the first cycle and regrowth. Chemical composition of forage (Table 1) was significantly different between periods in OM (89.4 vs 88.0% ; $P < 0.05$), Nx6.25 (15.1 vs 16.4 ; $P < 0.05$), NFE (45.5 vs 41.5 ; $P < 0.01$) and lignin level (9.7 vs 11.3 ; $P < 0.05$). These differences could be due either to the normal development and maturation of Gramineae or to seasonal changes in the botanical composition of the sward (Caputa, 1966; Ziliotto and Testolin, 1981). Table 1 includes the digestion coefficients and the nutritive values of the forages. Notwithstanding the differences in chemical composition, the digestibility coefficients of DM, OM, crude protein and NFE were similar in the two periods.

TABLE 1   Chemical composition, apparent digestibility coefficients and energy value of forage fed during digestibility trials

Period	Chemical composition		Digestibility coeff.(%)	
	Primary	Regrowth	Primary	Regrowth
Dry matter	14.3	14.9	60.3	60.8
Organic matter	89.4[a]	88.0[b]	62.6	63.3
N x 6.25	15.1[b]	16.4[a]	59.2	62.4
Crude fiber	25.1	25.7	61.3	61.3
N-free ext.	45.5A	41.5B	66.4	66.4
ADF	41.0	41.5	59.3A	54.0B
Hemicellulose	21.7	20.4	75.6B	89.7A
Cellulose	27.3	26.4	68.6[a]	64.2[b]
Lignin	9.7[b]	11.3[a]		
M.E. MJ/kg DM	8.82	8.81		
FUM/kg DM	0.74	0.72		

A, B: $P < 0.01$;   a, b: $P < 0.05$

Data in Table 1 also show differences in digestibility between the periods in fibrous components. In the second period a significant reduction of digestibility of ADF (54.0 vs 59.3% ; P < 0.01) and cellulose (64.2 vs 68.6% ; P < 0.05), was probably due to the different content of lignin in the forages; an increase in hemicellulose digestibility (82.7 vs 75.6% ; P < 0.01) was observed. Cellulose digestibility, calculated from Jarrige and Minson's (1964) equation using lignin content, gave values in good accordance with those observed in vivo. The nutritive value of forages (Table 1) estimated from the coefficients of digestibility and expressed in M.E. (Blaxter and Boyne, 1978) or in UFL (I.N.R.A., 1978) was similar in the two periods. In particular, the UFL content was in close accordance with that obtained using the equation of Andrieu et al. in I.N.R.A. (1978).

Table 2 reports the results of the grazing trial: data from two heifers were omitted. There were no important interactions between previous experience in grazing and grazing method, so only means for main effects are given. In the first period (0-14 d) the animals lost weight with greater losses in heifers not previously accustomed to graze. In the second period (15-55 d) daily gain in animals accustomed to grazing was significantly greater but following the 55th day no effect was noted. Grazing method did not effect daily gains over the whole trial. Forage disappearance on rotational grazing, measured after each grazing cycle, was 70-75% of herbage available before grazing, compared with 40-50% estimated in continuous grazing conditions.

Table 2   Effect of previous experience of grazing and of grazing method on liveweight of heifers at pasture

		Previous grazing experience		Grazing method	
		Accustomed	Not Accustomed	Rotation	Continuous
No. of heifers		9	9	9	9
Liveweight at turning out (20/5/81)					
	kg	291.3	353.6**	319.3	325.6
" " after 14 d (3/6) "		285.8	333.4*	306.9	312.3
" " " 55 d (14/7) "		305.4	342.6	320.1	327.9
" " " 77 d (5/8) "		310.7	345.8	324.7	331.8
" " " 163 d (30/10)"		337.9	366.0	-	-

CONCLUSIONS

Rotational grazing did not give any advantage in daily gain in comparison with continuous grazing but it allowed an increase in stocking rate from 1.5 head/ha to 5.5 head/ha. Chemical composition of native grass was slightly affected by period; in particular changes were observed in fibrous components and in Nx6.25. Apparent digestibility coefficients were low and differed between periods only for crude protein,ADF and celluloses.

REFERENCES

A.O.A.C. 1970. Official methods of analysis, XI ed. Association of Official Chemists, Washington, D.C.
Blaxter, K.L. and Boyne, A.W. 1978. J. agric. Sci., **90**, 47.
Caputa, J. 1966. Recherche agronomique en Suisse, 5 (3-4); 393.
Goering, H.K. and Van Soest, P.J. 1970. Forage fibre analysis. Agric. Res. Serv., United States Department of Agriculture, Jacket n. 387-598.
I.N.R.A. 1978. Alimentation des ruminants. Ed. I.N.R.A. Versailles 78000.
ISTAT 1982. Le regioni in cifre. Instituo Centale di Statistica, Roma.
Jarrige, R. and Minson, D.J. 1964. Annales de Zootechnie **13**, 117.
Ziliotto, U. and Testolin, R. 1981. Rivista di Agronomia, **XV**, 3-4, 143.

PREVENTIVE MEASURES TO CONTROL INTESTINAL PARASITES IN GRAZING YOUNG STOCK

D. Oostendorp[1], F.H.M. Borgsteede[2] and A. Kloosterman[3]

1. Research and Advisory Institute for Cattle Husbandry, Lelystad,
     Runderweg 6, 8219 PK, Lelystad, The Netherlands
2. Central Veterinary Institute, Department of Parasitology,Edelhertweg 15
     8219 PH, Lelystad, The Netherlands
3. Agricultural University, Department of Animal Husbandry, Marijkeweg 40,
     6709 PK, Wageningen, The Netherlands

INTRODUCTION

Intestinal nematode worms are a potential danger for young stock on all cattle farms. In spite of the knowledge of the life cycles of these parasites and the availability of anthelmintics there is a considerable loss because often the disease is diagnosed and treated too late (Kloosterman et al.,1981; Michel et al.,1981). For this reason it is very important to develop preventive measures to keep the level of worm infestation on a farm at a low and harmless level.

Grazing on aftermath

As an agricultural measure grazing on aftermath proved to be very successful in the Netherlands (Oostendorp and Harmsen, 1968). In this system calves are brought into the pasture after the first cut has been mown for silage or hay, and regrowth is available. Afterwards it is important to graze the calves in the period from May till September as much as possible on "clean" pasture. A condition for the application of this system is that fields are mown regularly for winter feed.

Strategic grazing and use of anthelmintics

On farms where there is no regular supply of aftermaths, e.g. farms with a very high stocking rate or farms with separate fields for grazing and cutting, a more strategic form of rotational grazing for the calves has to be applied (Michel, 1969, 1976; Borgsteede and Kloosterman, 1977). This has to be based on the knowledge of the influence of different factors on the development of the different worm species. With an average over-wintered infection and normal weather conditions under Dutch circumstances the more or less explosive appearance of infective larvae on the herbage (the mid-summer increase) does not take place until July. The calves have then to be moved to clean pastures from the paddocks where they have been grazed. Under favourable conditions these grazing measures will have to be combined with a strategic use of anthelmintics,e.g.in July and in the autumn.

Preventive use of anthelmintics

Where young stock are grazed in a rotational system without alternative cutting another possibility is to supply the animals with a preventive regular low dose of an anthelmintic during the first part of the grazing season. Systems in which this is realised by adding anthelmintics in drinking water, concentrates or licks break down on the fact that one cannot control the dose of each individual animal. A solution for this problem is presented by the Paratect bolus system (Jones, 1980).

In this system when cattle are turned out to pasture a bolus containing the anthelmintic morantel is administered by mouth and retained in the rumen of the animal. From this bolus the morantel is continuously released during a minimum period of 60 days. In this way the overwintered infective larvae are prevented from developing to adult worms and as a result no eggs will be deposited to infect the herbage which gives rise to reinfection.

In the Netherlands trials since 1979 proved the bolus to be effective in preventing parasitic gastroenteritis in calves and heifers (Borgsteede et al, 1981)

In the study presented here special attention was paid to the effects of the administration of a Paratect bolus to heifers with a different parasitic history. The research was carried out in co-operation with Mr. H. van Tarrij of Pfizer B.V.

Treatment groups

In 1981 one group of calves served as a control group. They were heavily infested with intestinal worms (maximum EPG 4850 on 30 June). The second group of heifers was treated with a Paratect bolus and showed only a very low level of egg output (maximum EPG 125 on 4 August). The third group of heifers was kept indoors as calves and fed with grass from always mown grassland. This group was not infested with intestinal worms. During the winter of 1981/1982 the heifers were housed and fed uniformly.

In 1982 a trial was carried out with these three groups of heifers with different parasitic histories. On 14 April,1982 each group of 14 animals was divided into two equal sub-groups each of 7 animals. Three sub-groups were put together as one group of 21 animals and grazed together; a Paratect bolus was administered to this group. The other group served as a a control.

In this way the following treatments were created:

Treatment 1981	Treatment 1982	Abbreviation
Control	Control	CC
Paratect bolus	Control	BC
Indoor feeding	Control	IC
Control	Paratect bolus	CB
Paratect bolus	Paratect bolus	BB
Indoor feeding	Paratect bolus	IB

Grassland management

The two groups of 21 heifers were rotationally grazed separately on 5.8 ha of grassland divided into 4 paddocks. At the start of the trial each paddock was divided into two for the two treatment groups to create paddocks with an equal parasitic history. This was checked by larval counts of grass samples. Grazing lasted from 14 April to 7 October. All through the season the grass supply was sufficient. On 28 May the surplus grass of one paddock was mown for silage.

Insemination

All heifers were artificially inseminated for the first time at an age of 15 months. If necessary the insemination was repeated three times. In group BB all animals came in calf. In the groups BC, CC and IC one heifer was not in calf, in group CB 2 heifers were not in calf and in group IB 3 heifers were not in calf.

Records

At the beginning of the trial the animals were weighed on two successive days and the Paratect boluses were administered to the treatment group. The animals were then weighed each 4 weeks. At each weighing blood samples were taken to analyse the pepsinogen level and the titer to parasites (Elisa test). Every two weeks faecal samples were taken from all animals for faecal egg counts and larval identification.

174

RESULTS

Liveweight gain

In Table 1 the growth results of 1981/82 are summarised.

TABLE 1   Weights and growth figures, calves 1981/82

	C	B	I
Weight 26/5/81 (kg)	94	94	94
Weight 29/10/81 (kg)	186	215	224
Weight 14/4/82 (kg)	310	333	348
Growth 26/5/81-29/10/81 (g/d)	590	776	840
Growth 29/10/81-14/4/82 (g/d)	743	707	743

In the first grazing period the average growth rates of the control group (C), the Paratect bolus group (B) and of the indoor feeding group (I) were 590, 776 and 840 g/d respectively. In the following winter period the growth of these three groups was practically equal, namely, 743, 703 and 743 g/d respectively. At the beginning of the second grazing season the weight of the control group was 310 kg, of the Paratect bolus group 333 kg and of the indoor feeding group 348 kg. In the second grazing season there were considerable differences between the 6 groups (Figure 1 and Table 2).

TABLE 2   Daily gain of heifers in 1982 (g/d)

	Treatment 1982		
Treatment 1981	B	C	Average
B	572	490	531
C	498	480	489
I	359	291	315
Average	476	414	445

The effect of the Paratect bolus was 476 - 414 = 62 g per day in favour of the bolus treatment. ($P<0.05$) (Figure 2)

This effect was independent of what happened with the animals in 1981 (no interaction). The animals which had been fed indoors during 1981 gained 195 g/d less, when they were grazed during 1982, than the average for animals (C and B) which had grazed during 1981.

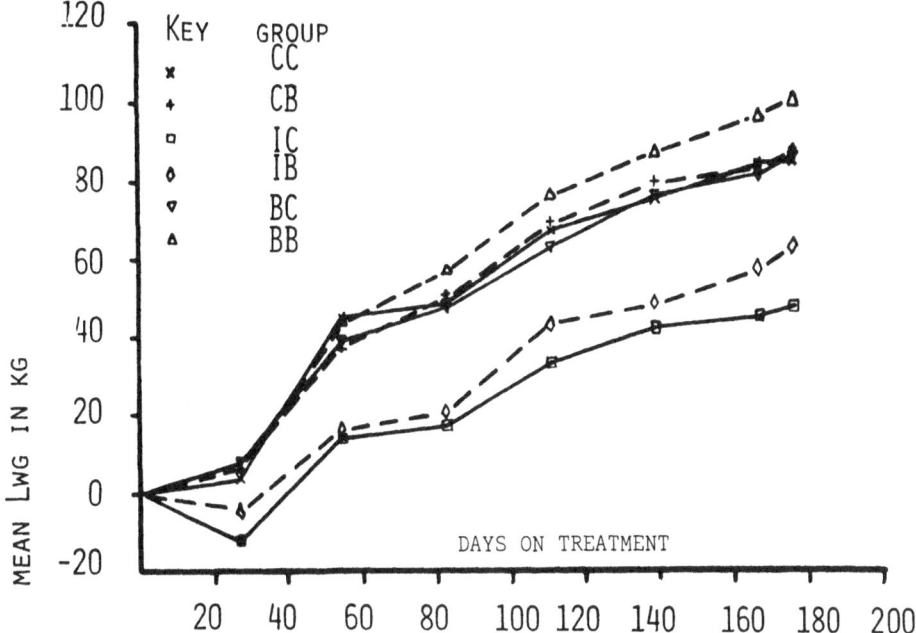

Fig.1 Heifer trial 1982, liveweight gain all groups

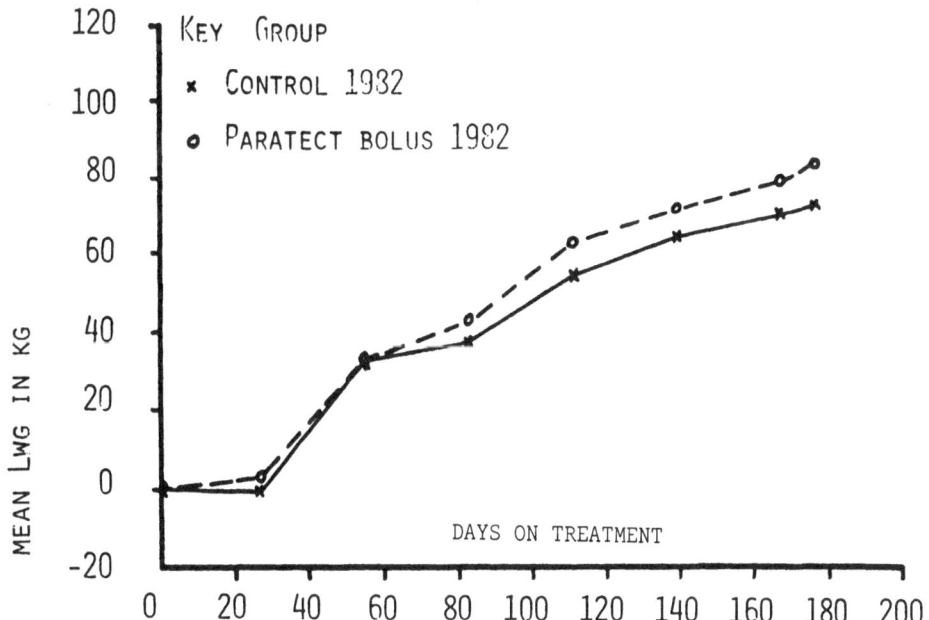

Fig.2 Heifer trial 1982, liveweight gain - combined results of
control and Paratect bolus groups

Larval counts and larval differentiation

It was striking that the EPGs of all groups stayed very low all through the season. Nevertheless, the larval count and the larval determination gave more details of the differences per group (Table 3)

TABLE 3   Larval counts (LPG) and larval differentiation in 1982

	CC	CB	BC	BB	IC	IB
Maximum LPG	11	6	19	4	37	33
Cooperia oncophora	-	-	+-	+	+	+
Ostertagia ostertagi	+	+	+	+	+	+
Trichostrongylus	+	+	+	+	+	+

In the two control groups of 1981 (CC and CB) the egg output remained very low all through the season. Cooperia oncophora was not present, so the heifers had obtained immunity to Cooperia oncophora. In the two Paratect bolus groups 1981 (BB and BC) the egg output also remained very low, especially in the group BB. There was a low egg output of Cooperia oncophora, which reduced to zero after June in the group BC. Immunity to Cooperia oncophora was quickly established. The egg output of the two indoor feeding groups in 1981 was significantly higher than the other 4 groups. However, the egg output was very low in comparison to the egg output of calves in the first grazing season. There was no immunity to Cooperia oncophora.

Pepsinogen level in the blood (Table 4)

The pepsinogen level in the blood is a measure of the infection of the mucous membrane of the abomasum by Ostertagia larvae.

At the beginning of the 1982 grazing season there was a big difference between the animals that had been on pasture in 1981 (C and B) and the housed animals (I). So, the indoor feeding group was not infected with Ostertagia in the first year. There was no difference between the control and the Paratect bolus group of 1981. Both groups were clearly infected with Ostertagia in their first year. During the grazing season 1982 there was a significant difference in pepsinogen level between the Paratect group and the control group ($P < 0.05$)

TABLE 4   Faecal samples and blood samples, 1982

Treatment 1981	Immunity to Cooperia oncophora (larval differentiation)	Infestation by Ostertagia ostertagi (pepsinogen level)	Titers to Cooperia and Ostertagia (Elisa test)
C	++	++	++
B	+−	++	++
I	−−	−−	−−

Elisa test (Table 4)

The Elisa test is a measure of the level of antibodies to parasites in the blood, thus reflecting the intake of larvae in the past. The results agree closely with the pepsinogen levels in the blood. At the start of the grazing season the titers of the indoor feeding group were significantly lower than those of the two groups that had been on pasture in 1981. This was analysed for the species Ostertagia and Cooperia. During the grazing season of 1982 the titers of the Paratect bolus group were consistently lower than those of the control group. In September these differences had disappeared, probably as a consequence of the end of the activity of the bolus.

CONCLUSION

The results of faecal and blood analyses lead to the conclusion that the restricted activity (±60 days) of the Paratect bolus leaves sufficient room for the building up of immunity. Indoor feeding of "clean" grass prevents a worm infestation but also prevents the building up of immunity. However, immunity is not absolute. The treatment of heifers with a Paratect bolus is not essential, but it can give an advantage in growth, depending on parasitological circumstances. In the trial of 1982 the average advantage was 62 g per animal per day. With heifers which have not been exposed to worm infestation during their first year extra care is required.

SUMMARY

It is important to develop simple preventive measures that keep worm infestation on a farm at a low harmless level. For this purpose grazing on aftermath has proved to be very successful in the Netherlands. Another approach is to supply the animals with a regular low dose of anthelmintic. This is offered by the Paratect bolus system. In 1982 a trial was carried out with three groups of 14 heifers with a different parasitic history to assess the efficacy of the bolus under different parasitological circumstances. It was concluded that the restricted activity ($\pm$60 days) of the bolus leaves sufficient room for the building up of immunity. Indoor feeding of "clean" grass prevented the building up of immunity. The treatment of heifers with a second Paratect bolus is not essential but can give an advantage in growth depending on parasitological circumstances.

REFERENCES

Borgsteede, F.H.M., and Kloosterman, A. 1977. Epidemiologie en profylaxe van trichostrongylose bij het rund. Tijdschr. Diergeneesk. **102** 1428

Borgsteede,F.H.M., Oostendoorp, D., van de Burg, W.P.J., Harmsen,H.E. and van Tarry, H. 1981. The Paratect bolus system in the prevention of gastro-intestinal nematode infection (English summary), Tijdschr. Diergeneesk. **108** 1255

Jones, R.M. 1980. A new method of control of gastro intestinal parasites in grazing calves. Proc. of the EEC Workshop on the epidemiology and control of Nematodiarisis in cattle. Copenhagen, February 4-6, 1980.

Kloosterman, A.,Borgsteede,F.H.M.,Jansen,J.,Koopman,J.J. and Oostendoorp,D. Farm management factors in relation to Trichostrongylosis in calves. 9th International Conference of WAAVP, Budapest, 1981, p.3 of Abstracts

Michel,J.F.The epidemiology and control of some nematode infections of grazing animals. Adv.Parasit. **7** (1969)211 and **14** (1976)355

Michel,J.F.,Hexham,J.P., Church,B.M. and Leech,P.K. 1981. Use of anthelmintics for cattle in England and Wales during 1978. Vet.Rec. **108** 252-258

Oostendorp,D.and Harmsen,H.E.1968. Agricultural control measures against intestinal parasites in cattle. Neth.J. Agric.Sci. **16** 177.

CONTINUOUS AND ROTATIONAL GRAZING FOR BEEF PRODUCTION[1]

L.Carlier, A. Andries and A. de Vliegher[2]

Government Plant Breeding Station, Burg. Van Gansberghelaan 109,B-9220, Merelbeke, Belgium

1. Research supported by the Instituut tot Aanmoediging van het Wetenschappelijk Onderzoek in Nijverheid en Landbouw (IWONL)
2. National Centre for Grassland and Green Fodder Research, Merelbeke, Belgium
   Communication R.v.P. N°482

INTRODUCTION

There is great interest in intensive continuous grazing, especially because of the saving in labour, but on the other hand there are some questions in connection with grass quality, animal health and animal production.

In view of the great interest in intensive continuous grazing with cows in the middle 1970s a comparison was made in Belgium between continuous and rotational grazing. This project also examined beef production from bulls, based on grass on a continuous grazing system.

MATERIALS AND METHODS

From 1977 to 1980, two comparable groups of young bulls started grazing each year early in May. One group grazed on a rotational system (8 plots each of 12.5 are) and the other group on a continuous system (1 ha)

In the rotational grazing system, 60 kg N/ha/grazing cycle was given and in the continuous grazing system 50 kg N/ha was applied every 3 weeks. Therefore differences in N-fertilization arose in some years in favour of the continuous system. The bulls were weighed monthly and when the grass-growth was insufficient the stocking rate was reduced. At the beginning of the grazing season the stocking rate was 9 bulls/ha (each approx 300 kg LW) decreasing to 6 bulls/ha at the end of the season. The bulls did not receive any supplement.

From 1979 the influence of techniques to combat stomach worms was investigated, partly by the use of thiabendazole (Merck, Sharp and Dohme), partly by the introduction of the Paratect bolus (Pfizer). Before the grazing period the bulls were vaccinated against lungworms with a product based on dictol (Philips Duphar).

In 1977 and 1978 the grass height was regularly measured on both systems and grass samples were taken for the determination of chemical composition.

RESULTS AND DISCUSSION

The data on stocking rate, N-fertilization, grazing period, starting-weight, daily liveweight gain and LWG/ha are given in Table 1 for both grazing systems.

TABLE 1   Intensive continuous grazing and rotational grazing with young bulls

Year	Grazing system (9 bulls/ha at start of season)	kg N /ha /yr	Grazing period days	Average starting weight kg	Average LW gain kg/d	Total kg/ha	Total animal-grazing days/ha
1977	continuous grazing untreated	250	127	301	0.690	702	1016
	rotational grazing untreated	240	127	300	0.790	798	1014
1978	continuous grazing untreated	300	150	287	0.564	741	1313
	rotational grazing untreated	300	150	288	0.691	895	1295
1979	continuous grazing treated	300	139	319	0.771	796	1032
	rotational grazing treated	240	139	322	0.753	886	1176
1980	continuous grazing treated	350	168	335	0.982	1169	1191
	rotational grazing treated	300	168	334	0.909	1193	1312
AVERAGE	continuous grazing	300	146	310	0.749	852	1138
	rotational grazing	270	146	310	0.786	943	1199

Over the 4 years of experiment (1977-1980) the individual growth was better on the rotational grazing system. The variation between the years however was great; in 1977 the grazing period was only 127 days (4 months) and in 1980, 160 days (5 months)

In a grazing system that is not balanced by fodder supplementation and where the animals are exclusively dependent upon the available quantity of grass, the weather conditions determining the grass growth are of great importance. Secondly, but no less important, is the intrinsic growth potential of the animals. Although the bulls for the 4 years of the experiment came from the same region (Ciney), the bulls of 1980 had obviously a higher growth capacity since the individual daily growth of the bulls was higher than in the previous years for both grazing systems.

The conclusion of our experiments seems to be that the rotational system must be preferred for growing animals, receiving no fodder supplementation during the grazing period, because this system allows 11% higher LWG production/ha, realised by a higher individual daily liveweight gain (5%) and a higher stocking rate (5%), the latter because of a more suitable grass availability.

TABLE 2 The effect of the treatments against stomach worms on the LW gain of young bulls in a continuous grazing system

Year	System	Grazing period days	Average starting wt kg	Average LW gain kg/d	LWG kg/ha	Total animal grazing days/ha
1979	continuous grazing untreated	139	319	0.771	787	1020
	continuous grazing treated	139	319	0.771	796	1032
1980	continuous grazing untreated	168	331	0.775	972	1254
	continuous grazing treated	168	335	0.982	1169	1191
1982	continuous grazing untreated	112	336	0.788	684	868
	continuous grazing treated	112	338	0.852	716	840
AVERAGE	continuous grazing untreated	140	329	0.778	814	1047
	continuous grazing treated	140	331	0.875	894	1021

The individual growth on the continuous grazing system can be improved by the application of efficient anthelmintics. Table 1, shows the higher daily liveweight gain of the animals in 1979 and 1980 when they were treated with thiabendazole than in 1977 and 1978.

The effect of an efficient treatment against stomach worms is still more clearly illustrated by Table 2, concerning the animal production and

Table 3, concerning the level of infection of the grass with infective larvae. In 1981 the infection of the untreated animals was so serious that they had to be taken off experiment. One of the animals had a count of 3400 eggs/g dung in July and died 10 days later. These animals were also affected by lungworms.

As far as the grass supply is concerned, Table 4 shows the grass length and availability and shows clearly that the grass height was the factor limiting grass uptake. When mown with a rotary mower to a 3cm stubble length, enough grass is apparently available for every bull but the grass is too short to be grazed easily.

TABLE 3   Infective larvae of stomach worms on grass of
the continuous grazing system - 1982

| | average number of larvae/kg grass | |
Date of sampling	Continuous grazing of untreated animals	Continuous grazing of treated animals
23/4	0	0
1/6	3 Cooperia	0
	1 Ostertagia	
7/7	50 Cooperia	0
	50 Ostertagia	
28/7	0	0
1/9	0	0

Reduced grass height and infection with stomach worms are the two main causes of a lower individual liveweight gain in a continuous grazing system with young cattle. The average number of eggs per gram (EPG) can be seen in Figure 1 for the two grazing systems.

In July-August the daily liveweight gains were lower on the untreated continuous grazed pasture. In the same period, the infection pressure with infective larvae of the stomach worms is also undoubtedly the highest. Countings on dung samples show that indeed in some experimental years the untreated bulls showed greater numbers of eggs per gram (EPG) (Table 5).

CONCLUSION

Intensive continuous grazing with young cattle, without an efficient treatment against stomach worms will result in lower individual liveweight

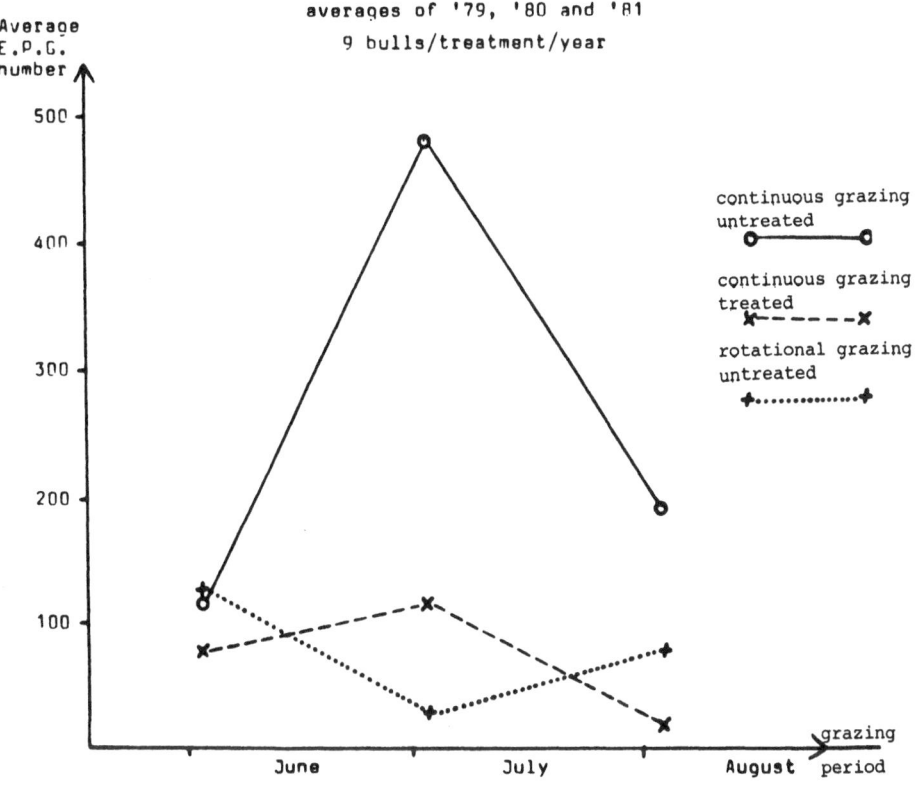

Fig. 1   Average EPG – number on continuous and rotational grazing
whether treated against stomach worms or not

gains and therefore in lower beef production per ha than in a rotational
grazing system, without a treatment against these worms. Depending upon the
degree of infection of the grass, an anti-worm treatment will result in a
less pronounced or a very positive influence on the individual liveweight
gain.

A continuous grazing system, not balanced by any form of fodder
supplementation, will have the disadvantage that the grass height may be
too short in some periods of the year to ensure a maximal uptake as is
possible in a rotational grazing system.   The unpredictability of grass
growth is the main cause of this situation.   To avoid this problem, a

TABLE 4   Average availability of grass/animal/day and the grass length on continuous and rotational grazing (at the beginning of grazing a plot)-1979

	Continuous grazing (1 ha)		Rotational grazing 8 plots of 0.125 ha	
Date	kg DM/a	length cm	kg DM/a	length cm
7/5	152	12.5	34	19.0
21/5	138	8.8	36	19.5
8/6	<u>36</u>	<u>4.8</u>	36	16.4
18/6	<u>23</u>	<u>4.2</u>	27	15.2
10/7	81	7.1	43	21.7
23/7	124	8.9	40	19.1
20/8	106	9.0	33	17.9
30/8	94	7.9	36	19.5

previous plan of the mowing percentage and the stocking rate should be made before the grazing season starts and adjustments should be made during the grazing period by increasing the pasture area or by decreasing the number of animals. On balance, it seems that the average stocking rate over the whole grazing season is somewhat lower on the continuous grazing than on the rotational grazing.

A third negative aspect of continuous grazing with young cattle is the need for a higher N-fertilization to ensure approximately the same grass availability. The labour saving effect of a continuous grazing system is outweighed by the negative aspects, considered above. Rotational grazing as a system for beef production on pasture is to be preferred above intensive continuous grazing.

TABLE 5   Average number of eggs per gram in dung of bulls during the grazing season

	Untreated continuous grazing			Treated continuous grazing			rotational grazing		
	June	July	August	June	July	August	June	July	August
1979	55	394	190	150	200	25	188	28	100
1980	160	360	89	17	50	11	56	17	44
1981	117	650	250	55	72	5	not determined		

MONENSIN-SODIUM AND LASALOCID-SODIUM AS GROWTH PROMOTERS FOR GRAZING YOUNG BEEF BULLS

Ch.V. Boucqué, L.O. Fiems, B.G. Cottyn and F.X. Buysse

National Institute for Animal Nutrition, Scheldeweg 68,
B-9231 Melle-Gontrode, Belgium
Communication No.533 of the Institute

INTRODUCTION

The contribution to beef production in Belgium expressed in carcass weight amounted to 7.8% from steers, 34.0% from bulls, 34.1% from cows and 24.1% from heifers in 1982 (INS, 1983). Bull beef production is mostly practised in a semi-intensive system. The inclusion of a pasture period is more profitable than continuous indoor feeding (Boucqué et al, 1978). An energy supplementation during this period is worthwhile for young calves (Fiems et al, 1979). This paper deals with the effect of monensin and lasalocid on the performance of young grazing bull calves.

MATERIALS AND METHODS

Two experiments were carried out with five-month old Belgian white-red bull calves to investigate the effect of monensin and lasalocid on animal performance and the grassland area used. The cattle were supplemented with 1 kg dried sugar beet pulp per day containing either 0 or 200 mg monensin in the first trial, and no additive, 250 mg lasalocid or 200 mg monensin in the second trial. During the first 14 days only 0.75 kg supplement was administered to all calves in the first trial and to the monensin fed calves in the second trial. The experiments lasted 168 and 154 days respectively. The animals were turned out on permanent grassland and rotational grazing was applied. The nitrogen dressing averaged 300kg per ha per year. The bull calves were weighed every 4 weeks. At the beginning and the end of the trial they were weighed on two consecutive days. Before the onset of the pasture period they were vaccinated against lungworms and IBR.

RESULTS AND DISCUSSION

The results of Trial 1 are given in Table 1. Monensin significantly increased daily gain from 0.65 to 0.79 kg ($P < 0.001$), an enhancement of 21.5%. A positive effect of monensin on daily gain had been found both with

186

ad lib supplementation, (Fiems et al, 1981) and with restricted supplementation on pasture (Potter et al, 1976; Rouquette et al, 1980). In our experiment the higher daily gain obtained with monensin was perceptible from the onset (Figure 1). Liveweight gain during the initial 28 days was significantly higher (P<0.001), in contrast to indoor finishing animals fed monensin (Burrin et al, 1982). Daily supplement intake was somewhat lower

TABLE 1   Effect of monensin on animal performance (± s$\overline{x}$)
(1st trial: summer 1980+1981+1982; 168 grazing days)

Monensin (mg/day)	0	200
Number of bull calves	46	46
Initial weight (kg)	158.2±2.2	158.5±2.1
Final weight (kg)	268.2±4.9	290.8±3.9
Liveweight gain (kg)		
– per day	0.65±0.02	0.79***±0.02
– per ha	1,146	1,364
Daily suppl. intake (kg)	0.98	0.97
Stocking rate		
– kg/ha	2,221	2,316
– animal/ha	10.4	10.3
Grazed area/animal (ha)	0.096	0.097

*** P < 0.001

for the monensin treatment, due to small refusals when the animals were moved to another paddock at the beginning of the grazing period. Generally the incorporation of monensin resulted in a slower intake. Although the additive resulted in a higher weight gain with a limited energy supplement the grazed area per animal was not markedly increased. Due to the higher daily gain on a similar area the liveweight gain per ha was 19.0% higher for the monensin group than for the control group. This may be explained by an altered rumen fermentation in favour of a higher propionic acid concentration (Cottyn et al,1983) and an increased digestibility with grazing cattle (Pond et al,1980). Monensin can therefore increase pasture carrying capacity. When we compare these results with earlier experiments where Belgian white-red bull calves were grazing in similar circumstances, but with or without ad lib energy supplementation, we observe that daily

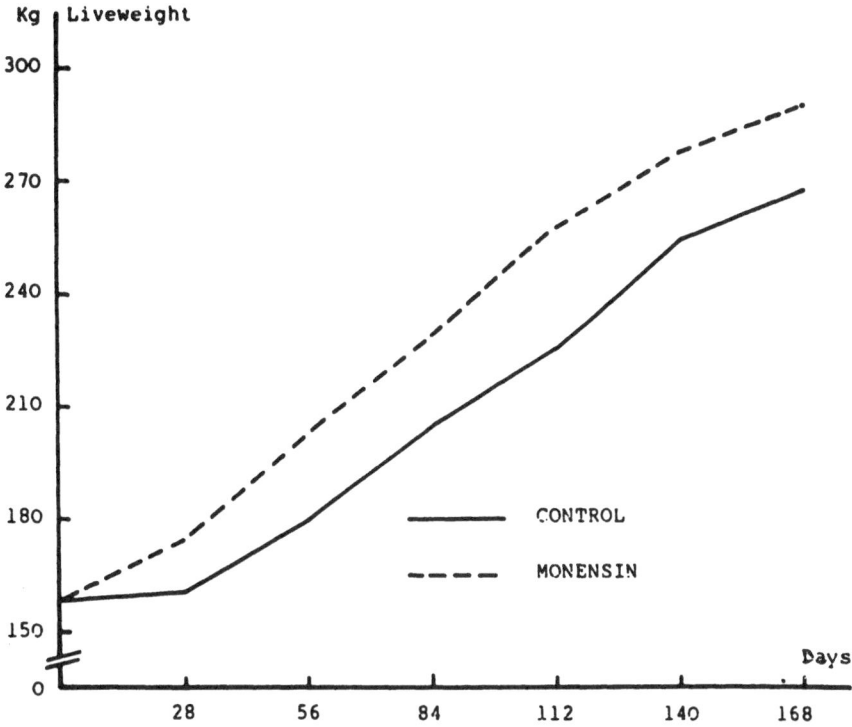

Fig. 1 Effect of monensin on liveweight gain of bulls on pasture

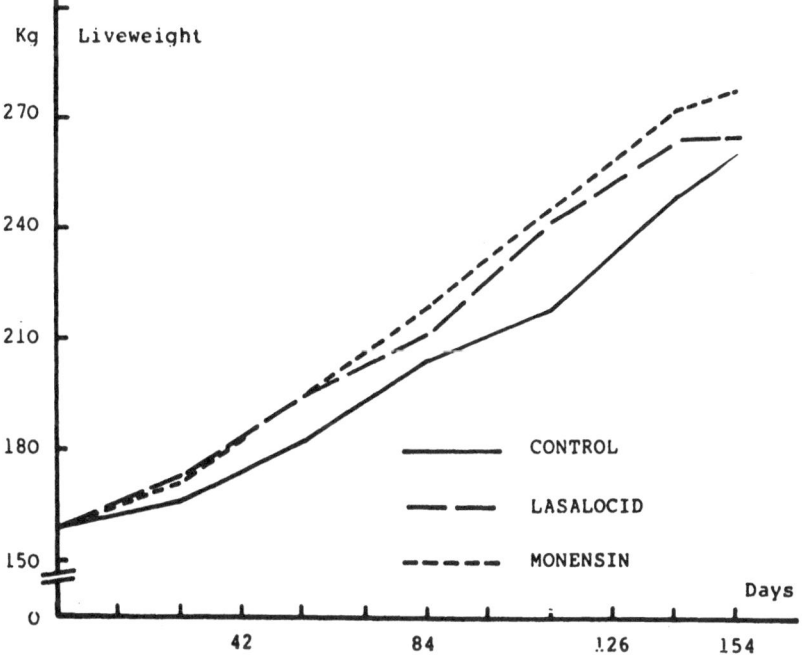

Fig. 2 Effect of lasalocid and monensin on liveweight evolution on pasture

gain was about the same when animals were either supplemented to appetite or received only 1 kg dried sugar beet pulp containing 200 mg monensin. These results are in Table 2.

TABLE 2   Effect of supplementation level and monensin

Dried beet pulp supplementation (kg/d)	0	1	1	ad lib
Monensin (mg/d)	0	0	200	0
Number of bull calves	46	46	46	44
Weight interval (kg)	159.6-218.6	158.2-268.2	158.5-290.8	162.5-278.1
Liveweight gain (kg)				
- per day	0.38	0.65	0.79	0.75
- per ha	383	1146	1364	1217
Suppl.intake (kg/d)	0	0.98	0.97	2.92
Stocking rate				
- kg/ha	1228	2221	2316	2319
- animal/ha	6.5	10.4	10.3	10.5
Grazed area/animal (ha)	0.154	0.096	0.097	0.095
Feed costs (BF)				
- per kg supplement	-	7.00	8.90	7.00
- per ha pasture	25000	25000	25000	25000
- per kg gain	65.2	32.2	29.3	47.9

The results of Trial 2 are presented in Table 3. Monensin significantly increased daily gain ($P<0.05$), while the growth rate with lasalocid was intermediate between the control and monensin fed calves. Lasalocid had a positive effect on liveweight gain during the main part of the grazing period, but during the last 14 days the difference in gain compared with the control group decreased, possibly because of reduced availability of grass (Figure 2). There are recent reports of a significantly improved gain by supplemented animals on pasture (Lomas, 1982; Spears and Harvey, 1982; Tanner et al., 1982). In these reports the optimum level of lasalocid was 200 mg per head per day, or less, while we administered a daily amount of 250 mg. In spite of the costs for incorporation of the additives the most favourable feed cost was obtained with monensin. With the lasalocid group the feed costs were less favourable than with the control group.

TABLE 3 Effect of lasalocid and monensin on animal performances ($\pm s\overline{x}$)
(2nd trial, summer 1982; 154 grazing days)

Additive Dose (mg/day)	Control -	Lasalocid 250	Monensin 200
Number of bull calves	18	19	20
Initial weight (kg)	160.0±4.2	159.9±2.9	159.8±3.0
Final weight (kg)	260.8±7.4	265.2±6.4	278.4±5.3
Liveweight gain (kg)			
- per day	0.65[a]±0.03	0.68[a]±0.03	0.77[b]±0.03
per ha	1,020	991	1,114
Daily supplement intake (kg)	1.00	1.00	0.98
Stocking rate			
- kg/ha	2,128	1,999	2,057
- animals/ha	10.1	9.4	9.4
Grazed area/animal (ha)	0.099	0.106	0.106
Feed costs (BF)			
- per kg supplement	7.00	9.00	8.90
- per ha.pasture	25,000	25,000	25,000
- per kg gain	35.2	38.3	33.6

a, b: values with unlike superscripts differ significantly ($P < 0.05$)

We can conclude that it is worthwhile to supplement young calves on pasture. Feeding 1 kg daily containing 200 mg monensin or 250 mg lasalocid resulted in an enhanced weight gain, especially with monensin, where the growth rate was similar to that of ad lib. supplemented animals, but with lower feed costs. The experiment with lasalocid will be repeated in 1983.

REFERENCES
Boucqué, Ch.V., Fiems, L.O., et Buysse,F.X. 1978. Influence de l'alimentation de veaux d'élevage au lait reconstitué ou au pis, et du système alimentaire, après la période d'élevage, sur les performances de taureaux à viande. Revue Agric., Brux. 31 :255-266
Burrin,D.G., Britton, R.A. and Brink,D.R. 1982. Effect of monensin in steers fed a high concentrate diet in initial 28 day adaptation and overall finishing performance. J. Anim.Sci. 55 , Suppl. I:412 (Abstr.)

190

Cottyn,B.G., Fiems,L.O., Boucqué,Ch.V., Aerts, J.V. and Buysse,F.X. 1983. Effect of monensin-sodium and avoparcin on digestibility and rumen fermentation. Z.Tierphysiol. Tiernährg. u. Futtermittelkde, **49** 277-286

Fiems.L.O.,Boucqué,Ch.V., et Buysse, F.X. 1979. L'effet d'une supplèmentation énergétique au cours de la période de pâturage sue les performances de génisses âgées de 5 à 11 mois. Revue Agric., Brux., **32** 1373-1381

Fiems,L.O., Boucqué,Ch.V., Cottyn, B.G.,de Brabander,D.L. et Buysse,F.X.1981.L'effet du monensin-sodium sur les performances de génisses broutardes. Revue Agric., Brux. **34** 899-909

Lomas, L.W. 1982. Effect of lasalocid sodium on gains of grazing steers. J. Anim. Sci., **55** , Suppl. I: 437 (Abstr.)

I.N.S. 1983. Statistiques agricoles Nr. 3.4 (Agricultural Statistics).Ministry of Economic Affairs, Brussels

Pond, K.R.,Ellis, W.C. and Telford, J.P. 1980. Monensin effects on intake,digestibility and rate of passage of ryegrass grazed by cattle. J. Anim. Sci. **51** Suppl. 1: 53 (Abstr.)

Potter, E.L., Cooley, C.O., Richardson,L.F., Raun, A.P. and Rathmacher, R.P. 1976. Effect of monensin on performance of cattle fed forage. J. Anim. Sci. **43** 665-669

Rouquette, F.M., Griffin, J.L., Randel, R.D. and Carroll, L.H. 1980. Effect of monensin on gain and forage utilization by calves grazing bermudagrass. J. Anim. Sci. **51** 521-525

Spears, J.W.and Harvey, R.W. 1982. Performance, ruminal and serum parameters of steers fed lasalocid on pasture.J. Anim.Sci. **55** Suppl.1:463 (Abstr.)

Tanner, J.W., Byers, F.M., Schake, L.M., Ellis, W.C., Schelling, G.T., Long, C.R. and May, R. 1982. Ionophore effects on growth rates of grazing stocker cattle. J. Anim. Sci. **55** , Suppl. I: 469 (Abstr.).

SUMMARY OF THE FINAL DISCUSSION

W. Holmes

General matters:

Contributors agreed that grass made a major contribution to the
nutrition of beef animals. Depending on the intensity of production, from
25-90% of the total diet may be provided from grass but higher proportions
from concentrates were usually associated with more rapid growth.   Later
maturing continental beef breeds generally required higher levels of
concentrate feeding.

There was a general view that to further cheapen production the
contribution of grass should be increased but the alternative view was also
expressed that, since grain production was likely to continue to expand in
Europe and to become cheaper, a greater use of grain might be economically
desirable. Although increased grain consumption was generally associated
with a decline in average carcase weight the use of higher levels of grain
with the larger breeds could maintain the level of meat production.

In contrast to the economic justifications for grain consumption
reference was also made to the social importance of maintaining rural
populations and encouraging livestock production from pasture in these
areas.

Another general matter of some importance was the probable decline in
the supply of calves suitable for beef production because of the static
demand for milk, the increasing use of Holstein type cattle and the
increased yield of milk per cow, leading to falling numbers of milk cows.

Genetic improvement

Important information was presented indicating a low correlation
between performance test and progeny test results for Friesian bulls in
Germany and suggesting that testing under intensive conditions might not be
appropriate where the normal product was older and of greater weight.
Methods of testing and selection of bulls for the various systems of beef
production were considered in detail. It was agreed that performance tests
should be conducted under similar circumstances to those under which the
commercial cattle would be produced.

Some doubt was expressed whether sophisticated genetic studies were
justified for beef production but it was generally agreed that if high
quality sires could be identified they could then be widely used both

to improve pure breeds at the top of the pyramid of breeding and in addition as cross breeding sires on dairy cattle. Analyses in Britain had shown a cost:benefit ratio of 1:2. The practical difficulties in the widespread use of artificial insemination in small herds were recognised.

Suckler beef production

Three papers demonstrated the considerable flexibility of the suckler cow and her ability to act as a reserve of nutrients. Data were provided indicating that she could store body reserves and then utilise them at a later stage in the production cycle and that this was often economic.

However it was agreed that the number of calves weaned per 100 cows, affected both by fertility and by calf mortality, was of vital importance and many of the investigations had not been of sufficient scale to indicate the effect of treatments on reproductive capacity.The possibility that in the long term multiple births might be achieved regularly from beef cattle was recognised as a possible contribution to a great increase in efficiency of meat production by these systems.

Questions were raised whether the suckler systems, essentially extensive and biologically inefficient could justifiably utilise the high nitrogen levels quoted in some of the experiments but it was claimed that these could be economically justifiable, although in favourable conditions white clover could supply much of the nitrogen required.

The point was also made that suckler cattle depending heavily on beef breeds were the major source of the high quality beef which will still command a premium in the market.

Beef production from dairy bred calves

It was recognised that in much of Europe the major source of calves for beef production would be pure bred bull calves from Friesian and Holstein cows with a limited use of beef cross calves from these breeds where cow longevity was long or where herds were large. In small herds the feasibility of cross breeding was limited since farmers were unwilling to risk having too few pure bred female replacements for the herd. Cross breeding was therefore likely to be important mainly in the larger herds in the United Kingdom, France and the Irish Republic. The probable increased use of extreme dairy type bulls would increase the difficulties of producing beef from dairy herds.

Some of the papers presented indicated how the considerable growth potential of beef animals could be realised. The adoption of rational pasture systems was essential. This usually involved grazing only half the area of pasture in the early part of the season,and conserving the other half, then using the total area for grazing in the later part of the season. Although there was little reference to the use of fertiliser nitrogen, its potential contribution to increased beef production from grass was accepted and was implicit in the papers on grassland planning. In addition where economic circumstances justified it, the use of supplementary feeds of grain or arable by-products might be justifiable to maintain rate of liveweight gain.

The consensus was that rotational systems of grazing were preferred particularly at high grazing pressures, as continuous stocking methods might reduce performance per animal and per hectare and increase the risk of helminth infection.

The papers on the utilisation of bulls for meat production confirmed that they did yield heavier and leaner carcases with more efficient utilisation of feed. Bull beef production is already widespread in some European countries and is likely to expand in others,for example France. However problems of behaviour, safety and meat quality remain and require further study and in Britain a combination of farmer, butcher, welfare and consumer considerations is likely to militate against the widespread production of bull beef.

The use of feed additives such as monensin sodium or lasalocid sodium to increase the rate of gain of beef animals, particularly where they were offered in association with lower quality diets indoors or on pasture, provided another method of increasing the rate of gain of beef animals.

The use of some anabolic agents is already banned in some countries. Divergent views were expressed, one that they should be universally banned, the other that they were better permitted but under strict control.

The control of health particularly of worm infestations was essential. This could often be achieved by methods of good husbandry and the use of clean grazing systems but strategic dosing with anthelmintics and the use of slow-release methods of administration could be useful in some circumstances.

With regard to techniques interesting information on the interaction of pasture supply and supplements on feed intake was provided and recent equipment for the automated recording of grazing behaviour was also described.

The future

Turning to the future it was considered that the demand for beef would be maintained in the richer countries, but it was important that greater consistency in beef quality should be achieved. By the nature of the product there was obviously a range of meat quality within the beef animal,but the presentation of beef to the consumer can be improved by the modification of butchering practices. With current British practices relatively small carcases are required to achieve high quality, but in French practice the skilled cutting of large carcases still yields satisfactory products.

Finally it was agreed that the many factors contributing to efficient beef production could be assembled in systems programmes and that while there might be many individual studies of the sectors of beef production systems it was necessary for them to be assembled into a comprehensive system analysis from which to develop effective advisory procedures. Although detailed systems analysis is extremely complex its presentation to the farmer need not be so.

List of participants

Dr.C.Beranger, Laboratoire de production de viande bovine, Centre de
   Recherches Zootechnique et Vétérinaire de Theix-INRA-63122,Ceyrat,FRANCE
Professor J.M. Bienfait, Faculté de Médicine Vétérinaire, Rue des
   Vétérinaires 45, B-1070, Brussels, BELGIUM
Dr. R.C. Campling, Department of Agriculture, Wye College (University of
   London), Ashford, Kent, UK
Dr. D.M.B. Chestnutt, Agricultural Research Institute, Hillsborough,
   Co. Down, UK
Mr. J. Connell, Commission of the European Community,200 Rue de la Loi,
   B-1049, Brussels, CEC
Mr.S. Curran, Agricultural Research Institute, Dunsinea, Castleknock,
   Co. Dublin, IRELAND
Dr..B.G. Cottyn, National Institute for Animal Nutrition,Scheldeweg 68,
   B-9231, Melle-Gontrode, BELGIUM
Dr.A.de Vlieger,Government Plant Breeding Station,Burg van Gansberghelaan
   109, B-9220, Merelbeke, BELGIUM
Dr. M.J. Drennan, The Agricultural Institute, Grange, Dunsany, Co. Meath,
   IRELAND
M. A. Faucon, ITEB, 149 Rue de Bercy, F-75595, Paris, FRANCE
Dr. J. Gibson, Animal Breeding Research Organisation, West Mains Road,
   Edinburgh UK
Dr. M. Gielen, Faculté de Médicine Vétérinaire, Rue des Vétérinaires 45,
   B-1070, Brussels, BELGIUM
Dr. H. Glover, East of Scotland College of Agriculture, Bush Estate,
   Penicuik, Midlothian, UK
Dr. F.J. Harte, The Agricultural Institute, Dunsany, Co. Meath, IRELAND
Dr. G. Hof, Agricultural University 6708, PM Wageningen,NETHERLANDS
Professor W. Holmes, Department of Agriculture, Wye College (University of
   London), Ashford, Kent UK
Professor H.J. Langholz, Institute of Animal Husbandry and Genetics,
   Albrecht-Thaer-Weg 1, 3400 Gottingen, GERMANY
Professor L.'t Mannetje, Agricultural University, 6709, PM Wageningen,
   NETHERLANDS
Dr.J.A.C. Meijs, Institute for Livestock Feeding and Nutrition Research,
   (IVVO), Runderweg 2, PO Box 160, 8200 AD Lelystad, NETHERLANDS
M F.Menissier,Station de Génétique quantitative et appliquée, Centre de
   Recherches Zootechnique et Vétérinaire-INRA_78350,Jouy-en-Josas,FRANCE
M D.Micol,Laboratoire de production de viande bovine, Centre de Recherches
   Zootechnique et Vétérinaire de Theix, 63122 Ceyrat, FRANCE
Mr. W.E.Murphy, Agricultural Institute,Johnstown Castle, Wexford,IRELAND
Mr. J. Noble, ADAS, Government Offices, Brooklands Avenue, Cambridge UK
Dr. D. Oostendorp, Research and Advisory Institute for Cattle Husbandry,
   Runderweg 6, 8219 PK Lelystad, NETHERLANDS
Dr. D.F. Osbourn, Grassland Research Institute, Hurley, Maidenhead,Berks UK
Dr.M.O'Sullivan,The Agricultural Institute,Johnstown Castle,Wexford,IRELAND
Dr. M. Pinosa, Istituto di Produzione Animale, Università degli Studi,
   33100 Udine, ITALY
Professor W.F. Raymond, High Walls, Pinkneys Lane, Maidenhead, Berks, UK
Mr. J.R. Southgate, Meat & Livestock Commission, PO Box 44, Queensway
   House, Milton Keynes MK2 2EF,UK
Mr.A.W. Spedding, Meat & Livestock Commission, PO Box 44, Queensway House,
   Milton Keynes MK2 2EF, UK
Dr.I.Wright, Hill Farming Research Organisation,Bush Estate, Penicuik,
   Midlothian, UK.